Sudden Death in Infancy

Sudden Death in Infancy

The 'cot death' syndrome

BERNARD KNIGHT

MD, BCh, FRCPath, DMJ(Path)

Barrister-at-Law, Professor of Forensic Pathology,
Welsh National School of Medicine,
University of Wales, Cardiff
Honorary Consultant Pathologist, Cardiff Royal Infirmary
Home Office Pathologist

———

With a Foreword by
The Countess of Limerick MA

Executive Chairman of the
Welfare and Information Committee, and
Vice-Chairman of
The Foundation for the Study of Infant Deaths

faber and faber

First published in 1983
by Faber and Faber Limited
3 Queen Square London WC1N 3AU
Filmset by Wilmaset, Birkenhead, Merseyside
Printed in Great Britain by
Redwood Burn Ltd., Trowbridge, Wiltshire
All rights reserved

British Library Cataloguing in Publication Data

Knight, Bernard
Sudden death in infancy.
1. Infants–Mortality
I. Title
618.9   RJ59

ISBN 0-571-13066-6

Library of Congress Cataloging in Publication Data

Knight, Bernard.
Sudden death in infancy.

Bibliography: p.
Includes index.
1. Sudden death in infants. I. Title. [DNLM:
1. Sudden infant death. WS 430 K69s]
RJ59.K58   1983   618.92   82–25501
ISBN 0-571-13066-6

Contents

Foreword by the Countess of Limerick

The sudden unexpected death of a baby is the most common but least understood kind of death among babies aged between one week and two years. It is also one of the most distressing and baffling tragedies with which officials, health professionals and relatives are involved. It is not a new problem but one which has become more prominent as other fatal conditions in infancy have been reduced or prevented. It is probably only over the past decade that the public have really become aware of them. But so long as the reasons for these tragedies are little understood, it is easy for myths and misconceptions about their cause to survive.

Confusion sometimes arises over what is meant by a cot death (crib death) since formerly the terms were used to describe any unexpected infant death for which there are many different reasons. Recently, these terms have come to be confined to the unexpected deaths which remain unexplained or only partially explained at post-mortem, referred to medically as sudden infant death syndrome.

Sudden infant deaths are the third largest problem of all infant mortality after perinatal conditions and congenital anomalies. The number is substantially greater than the number of children under 15 who are killed on the roads, and the incidence is now higher among live-born children than the incidence of Down's syndrome, cystic fibrosis, spina bifida or any form of cancer in children under 15 years. Sudden infant deaths are important not only for numerical reasons but also because of the profound psychological impact they have on the bereaved parents.

The death of a child is a heart-rending tragedy in most circumstances. When it occurs suddenly, unexpectedly and for no obvious reason in an apparently normal infant whose symptoms of illness, if any, were considered trivial, the shock, guilt and bewilderment are traumatic and long-lasting.

Professor Knight's most readable book is therefore particularly welcome for a wide range of readers. He looks at the problem of sudden infant deaths in historical perspective and describes what in the light of recent studies is known about the babies and families to whom these tragedies occur; he explains the reasons for the coroner's enquiry and discusses many of the numerous hypotheses which have been put forward. As Professor Knight himself points out, it may be that in years to come there will be a much clearer understanding of how and why these babies die.

Most importantly Professor Knight makes many helpful suggestions about how officials can perform their legal responsibilities in a tactful manner and how members of the medical and nursing professions can help parents by giving informed support. There are other caring professionals such as ministers of religion, social workers, psychiatrists and also the families' relatives and neighbours who do so much to comfort the bereaved parents and their surviving children. They also need to understand what is known about these tragedies.

This book will be of value and interest not only to parents whose baby dies suddenly, and their relatives and friends, but also to officials such as the coroner, coroners' officers, police, ambulance and accident and emergency staff, funeral directors, as well as doctors, health visitors, midwives and nurses, ministers of religion, child care organisations and others who may be involved.

Professor Knight is both a barrister and pathologist; he is also a very humane and compassionate person who has actively used his professional knowledge and personal experience to focus public attention on this major problem of child health and to improve the way the deaths are managed. He is much too modest about his own role in persuading national and international institutions to recognise sudden infant deaths as a natural registrable cause of death; and with his wife in giving reassurance and information to bereaved parents by founding the British Guild for Sudden Infant Death which has happily merged with the Foundation for the Study of Infant Deaths.

Sylvia Limerick

The Foundation for the Study of Infant Deaths
5th Floor, 4 Grosvenor Place
London, SW1X 7HD

Author's preface

> What greater pain can mortals bear than this;
> To see their children die before their eyes?
>
> Euripides 480–406 BC

The sudden, unexpected death of an apparently healthy baby is probably the most poignant and devastating event that can overtake a young couple – yet in Western society it is also the most common kind of infant death after the first week of life.

The toll of infant life in Europe, North America and Australasia is known to run into many thousands each year but, until about two decades ago, sudden infant death was virtually unknown not only to the general public but to most of the medical profession, except as a series of misconceptions and misapprehensions that lingered in an almost medieval aura of neglect and ignorance.

It has taken bereaved parents, rather than doctors, to revolutionise this situation in the last few years. On both sides of the Atlantic, voluntary groups forced this greatest killer of babies to the attention of the medical and health care professions.

This book attempts to set out, in a comprehensible way, the current state of affairs concerning all aspects of 'cot' or 'crib' deaths. It is directed mainly at parents, non-specialist doctors, and all health and social workers – professional and voluntary – in the front line of supportive action which is so vital to keep newly-bereaved parents out of the despair which was their lot until recent times.

The book is not a medical or scientific treatise on the pathology of sudden infant death – others are better qualified to produce such a work – but one chapter is devoted to current ideas about the causes of the sudden infant death syndrome. Though recent and somewhat controversial attempts to devise some form of prevention are also described, the text mainly concerns its impact on the family –

especially the mother – and the need for and the content of support and counselling to alleviate its worst effects.

> Give sorrow words; the grief that does not speak
> Whispers the oe'r-fraught heart
> And bids it break
>
> *Macbeth*, IV. iii. 209

Acknowledgements

I am indeed grateful to Lady Limerick for kindly writing the Foreword to this book: it allows me the opportunity to thank her not only for her enthusiastic support, but also for the devoted work she performs on behalf of the Foundation for the Study of Infant Deaths.

My profound thanks are due also to Miss P. A. Downie FCSP, Medical and Nursing Editor, Faber and Faber, for her own expert counselling and forbearance in the preparation of this book.

Figures 2, 4, 7 and 8 are based on figures collected by Dr Preben Geertinger; Figure 3 is based on figures published by the Registrar-General of Births and Deaths: to both I extend my thanks.

The leaflets on pages 109–11, 115–17 and 155–8 are reproduced in full by permission of the Foundation for the Study of Infant Deaths.

B.K., 1982

Note for readers in the United States

The term 'cot death' is used throughout,
though the author well knows that in your
country the term would be 'crib death'.

1 · What is it?

Whenever doctors write about some disease or condition, they always give references to articles from medical journals, especially its first description. For instance, the main features of the 'battered child syndrome' were first published by a Dr Caffey in an American journal of radiology in the 1950s and 1960s.

To find the original literature on cot death, however, we need not refer to the *Lancet* for 1926 or the *Journal of the American Medical Association* for 1942. We have to look much further back in time – in fact, we need to take down a copy of the Bible.

There, in the Old Testament, we can turn to Chapter III of the First Book of Kings and read the judgement of Solomon about the death of a baby, which sounds uncommonly like the sudden infant death syndrome. Solomon had to decide the parentage of a surviving infant when two women came to him both claiming to be its mother. The reason that there were two mothers and only one child was that the other child 'had been overlain in the night'. As we shall see, overlaying was the classical belief for the cause of cot death until very recently. The only point against the Old Testament tragedy's being a true cot death was that the child was only three days old, which is too young for a true sudden infant death – but perhaps errors in translation may account for the discrepancy.

Solomon's case was about 3000 years ago and it seems very likely that sudden deaths have been occurring in infants for as long as man has existed.

Another classic description occurs in a medieval book by a Welsh priest, Giraldus Cambrensis. In the year A D 1188, he accompanied Archbishop Baldwin on a recruiting campaign for the Third Crusade. At Cardigan, West Wales, the Archbishop preached his sermon and called for volunteers for the Holy War. A number of men came forward, but the wife of one grabbed his cloak and prevented him from 'taking the Cross'. Three nights later, she woke up suddenly after a frightening dream and, on falling asleep again, accidentally smothered her infant boy of whom Giraldus said 'who with more affection than prudence she had brought into her own bed'. Once again we see this misunderstanding about overlaying which has persisted for thousands of years and has caused so much unnecessary anguish to mothers.

So cot death has always been with us and apparently it does not affect the human race only. Veterinary surgeons report that it also occurs in animals, including pigs and guinea-pigs, some of whose offspring die inexplicably in a similar way.

A definition of cot death

For a long time, confusion reigned about what states were meant when the term 'cot death' was used. To make the matter clear and to exclude the previous confusion with other types of infant death, a working definition has now been accepted. This does not help us to understand the cause, but at least it establishes a common baseline from which to begin. At one of the early international conferences on the topic, in Seattle, USA, in 1969, the matter of nomenclature – which was rather indeterminate in the previous Seattle conference in 1963 – was discussed and, from that time, almost all people involved in surveys and research have accepted the label 'Sudden Infant Death Syndrome', now commonly abbreviated to SIDS. A definition of SIDS was put forward at Seattle and widely accepted. This was devised by Dr J. Bruce Beckwith of Seattle, one of the pioneer workers in the USA, who proposed that the definition should be: 'The sudden death of any infant or young child which is unexpected by history and in which a thorough post-mortem examination fails to demonstrate an adequate cause for the death'.

The words 'infant or young child' were later refined to an age range of between two weeks to two years though, very occasionally, a child under two weeks has to be called a SIDS because the rest of the definition fits the death.

For long before this definition was worked out, a more colloquial description was in use both by doctors and the public. This was 'cot death' in Britain and 'crib death' in North America. These were very convenient and descriptive terms for the tragedy, but not as accurate as the full SIDS definition, for they meant only that an infant was found dead in its sleeping place. Though virtually all SIDS are cot or crib deaths, not all cot or crib deaths are true SIDS; some babies die in their sleeping places of specific diseases which are not the unexplained condition of Dr Beckwith's definition. This is not mere splitting of hairs or playing with words, as will be seen when we come to talk about the possible causes of SIDS. Where scientific accuracy is not an issue, however, the use of the terms cot or crib deaths will be assumed by almost everyone to refer to the true sudden infant death syndrome.

This leads us to the last point concerning definitions, the meaning of 'syndrome', which confuses many people. It is really an alternative to a disease, in the medical sense of the word. A 'disease' is a definite entity, usually due to a single abnormality and of which the cause is usually known. For example, smallpox is a disease, always due to a single cause, infection from a virus. There are many well-recognisable illnesses, however, which have a typical group of symptoms, but where the mechanism and cause is not known. SIDS is one of these, for it is now generally accepted that the sudden, unexpected death of a young infant in its sleeping place is such a common and characteristic happening that there have to be some common factors involved. This is not to say that all cot deaths have the same cause – almost certainly they do not – but the mercilessly repetitive circumstances are so similar that it cannot be a chance, random coming-together of characteristics like age, time, season, sleep etc., but must have enough of a common pattern to become a specific collection of symptoms justifying the label 'syndrome'. In other words, the cases are so repetitive in nature that there is some common thread, but not enough to warrant calling it a 'disease'.

How big is the problem?

For the next few sections, we have to look dispassionately at the whole subject of SIDS, trying to put aside the intensely tragic circumstances of each case. We have to look at the over-all picture, in other words study the epidemiology or

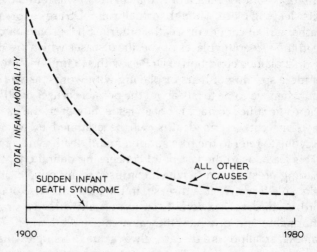

Fig. 1 Mortality rates for infants, 1900–80, showing the decline for all causes *except* SIDS which remains constant

how the condition fits into the whole spectrum of fatal childhood conditions and how it attacks various sections of the population at large.

One reason why both medical and public interest in the sudden infant death syndrome has increased so dramatically during the last 15–20 years is that it has become very apparent that SIDS is one of the major problems in infant mortality. This new awareness naturally applies far more in the developed countries than among those of the Third World because of the lower total infant mortality rate and the far

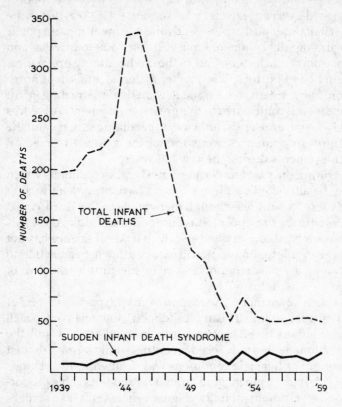

Fig. 2 The pattern in Copenhagen, Denmark, of post-neonatal mortality (2–11 months of age) over the 20 years spanning the last war. Even though 'all other causes' were worse during the occupation, they fell dramatically afterwards. SIDS, however, showed no significant variation

better statistical records in advanced countries. In these countries, from the latter part of the nineteenth century and especially after the turn of the twentieth century, infant mortality dropped dramatically – and continued to do so until after the Second World War, when the level tended to flatten out. In Figures 1 and 2 it can be seen that from the year 1900, for example, there was a rapid fall in infant mortality in

Europe and North America, but that the decrease, once it reached a certain level, failed to continue. This was due to the fact that the almost explosive advances in medicine and public health rapidly conquered most diseases due to external and environmental factors. Care of the mother during pregnancy, better child-birth facilities, better maternal and infant nutrition, better infant welfare and new methods of treating infant diseases all contributed to this great improvement. Advances in hygiene, antisepsis, antibiotics, paediatric surgery and the control of epidemics were among the greatest of medical achievements during the last 100 years.

During the past few decades, most of the conditions which can be alleviated by these methods have been dealt with in advanced countries – though many parts of the Third World are still in the same position as Europe in the Middle Ages. This leaves a hard core of diseases which medical science has not yet been able to conquer; it will require a much greater effort to achieve a smaller improvement in the future – the law of diminishing returns.

When infant mortality was rampant, with perhaps a third of all infants dying in early childhood, the relatively small contribution of SIDS was hardly noticed – this is still the situation in less advanced countries. But when the vast majority of treatable conditions was dealt with, the obvious SIDS became a much more prominent and noticeable proportion of total infant mortality. Figure 1 shows SIDS as a straight line on the graph, because it has not been modified – as far as we can tell – by any external influences. Although this is merely a diagram actual figures are available for Denmark (Fig. 2).

In highly-advanced countries, SIDS is now the most common single cause of death after the perinatal period (first seven days of life) and in some places it is more common than *all other causes of death combined at the age of three months*.

How many cot deaths occur?

Estimates of the true incidence of SIDS vary considerably from place to place and from researcher to researcher. Much of the variation is due to differences in the methods of compiling statistics. Because of the variation in the names given to SIDS by different doctors (see p. 16), it is still difficult for researchers to identify all cases in a given area. Indeed, until recently, there was no such category provided in the International Classification of Diseases, the official list published by the World Health Organisation: only in 1979 was a coding number alloted (798–0). It was therefore impossible to get accurate statistics, as certifying habits vary so much from country to country and even from doctor to doctor in the same country.

Matters are rapidly improving in this respect and our present knowledge is increasing about the true incidence of the condition. At the present time, most of our knowledge is based on a large number of smaller series of SIDS compiled by paediatricians and pathologists who have had a special interest in infant death. In addition, recent years have seen a number of more ambitious research schemes in Britain, America, Australia and Scandinavia, contributing greatly to our knowledge of how many cases actually occur.

Estimates for Britain some years ago varied between 1500 and 3000 per year. At that time, in the 1960s, the birth-rate was higher than at present, so that currently it is thought that between 1000 and 2000 deaths occur each year. With regard to numbers in England and Wales, some interesting data were published by the Registrar-General in December 1980 (Fig. 3). This showed that in 1978 – the last year for which, at the time of publication, he had figures – there were 971 SIDS reported to him on death certificates. This number came in a year in which there were almost 600 000 live births; seven years earlier, there were only 489 SIDS certified in almost 800 000 births.

These figures, as the Registrar-General himself pointed out, carried two major inaccuracies; first, they by no means indicated all the SIDS occurring in England and Wales, because they came only from death certificates which actually had 'sudden infant death' written upon them. It is well known that many doctors do not use the term, but employ a

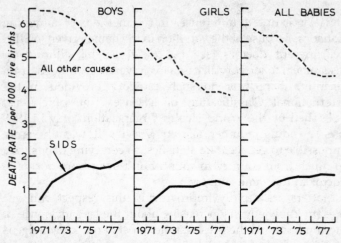

Fig. 3 The pattern of post-neonatal deaths in England and Wales 1971–78, showing the overall improvement but a worsening of SIDS (due to the increased use of the term SIDS on death certificates). Note that there is a slight, but constant, excess in boys (Registrar-General's figures)

wide variety of other causes, many obviously quite far from the truth in terms of pathology. The second fault also stems from this, in that there has *not* been a huge rise in SIDS between 1971 and 1978, as the figures suggest (from a rate of 0.62 per 1000 in 1971 to 1.63 in 1978). It is due, of course, to the marked increase in awareness of doctors of the existence of the sudden infant death syndrome, so that increasingly they are using it on certificates. If one went back to, say, 1950, the 'official' SIDS rate in England would be zero, because no one had heard of the term then – it had not been devised.

The 1980 statistics also show that there was a definite excess of boy victims over girls and also that the peak age for SIDS was between two and three months, perhaps a little younger than some other surveys indicate. The 1978 rate of 1.63 per 1000 is lower than other figures elsewhere, almost certainly due to under-reporting; if they are corrected to about 2 per 1000 and the victims in Scotland and Ireland added, it can be seen that approaching 2000 deaths in the whole British Isles can be attributed to SIDS.

In the United States, it was said in 1960 that there were approximately 6000 crib deaths, though one very well-known paediatrician alleged in 1966 that there may have been between 15000 and 25000 cases each year.

As we shall see later, the rate differs according to geography and social conditions, but at the time of writing most authorities in Northern Europe, North America and Australasia would agree that about one child in every 500 born alive will suffer a cot death. This is the same as saying that the incidence is about 2 per 1000 as it is conventional to state death rates of this order of magnitude in terms of cases per 1000 population, the population here being live births. This rate of 2 per 1000 is a generalisation and considerable variations occur on both sides. Some areas report a lower incidence, others a substantially higher rate. For instance, in American service families living in Germany, the rate was at one time as high as 1 per 160 live births.

To illustrate the results from a number of local surveys, an investigation in the author's own city of Cardiff (Wales) between 1965 and 1977 revealed an overall rate of 2.1 per 1000, just about the accepted average. In Newcastle-upon-Tyne in 1974–5, the rate was 3.7 per 1000, but this was in an area with a high over-all infant mortality (post-perinatal) of over 11 per 1000 births.

In the USA, the rate for Long Island is quoted as 1.46 per 1000, which is rather lower than average. In North Carolina and Nebraska, there were 2.06 and 2.55 per 1000 respectively. The figures for North Carolina were an average for different ethnic groups – significantly, the white infants had a SIDS rate of only 1.23, while negro babies had 3.73 and Indian infants no less than 6.56 per 1000, almost certainly a reflection of social rather than racial causes.

That differences in nomenclature alter the figures is seen from a Tasmanian survey, where, though the stated SIDS rate is 2.94 per 1000, if other deaths called 'chest infections' – but which most probably are almost all SIDS – are included, the rate jumps to almost 4, one of highest recorded in an advanced country with a Caucasian population.

Whereas Tasmania is a high incidence area, Israel's rate is said to be only 0.67. Another very low-rate country is Finland, which – though climatically very different from Israel – is renowned for its excellent child health care services and, as suggested by research in Sheffield and other centres, these in themselves seem to lower the SIDS rate. Other countries with low cot death rates, below 1 per 1000, include Sweden and the Netherlands.

Averaging all these figures in developed countries, it would seem reasonable to agree that about 1 SIDS per 500 live births constitutes the general incidence. However, we have to look much more closely at this overall rate and explore certain sections of the infant population to see whether any particular sections are more or less at risk.

AGE

The age of the infant victims is a very important factor for SIDS attacks a quite specific group of children in relation to their time since birth. Sudden infant deaths do not occur in the new-born. Though there is a substantial mortality in the neonatal and perinatal period (up to seven days after birth) this is not the time during which SIDS strikes them. Very occasionally, a week-old babe will die in circumstances identical with typical SIDS and the post-mortem examination fails to reveal any other reason for the death – so by exclusion the tragedy may be labelled as a cot death. But this is rare and the very young infant is unlikely to suffer a cot death within the first month of life. This fact is another argument against the rearguard action of those who still try to maintain that mechanical suffocation is the cause of SIDS. We shall look into this later on, but it seems obvious that the long-held idea that cot deaths were due to overlaying or suffocation by pillows or bedclothes fails to explain why most cases occur in babies of three to six months of age. Surely these more robust infants would be less at risk than the tiny tots of a few days or a week or two if asphyxia from bedclothes was the answer?

The great majority of cot deaths take place between the second and sixth months (Figs. 4 and 5), though there is tapering-off at either end of this range. At one of the early International Conferences on SIDS held at Seattle, it was agreed that the 'official' age range was between two weeks and two years, but this decision sets the extreme limits – apart from the maverick case at about a week. Very few take place after seven to nine months and those occurring in the second year are very rare indeed.

The risk period follows a typical curve, as shown in Figure 4, with a central peak at about two to four months and diminishing slopes on either side. This danger period at about two to three months is very real – one survey showed

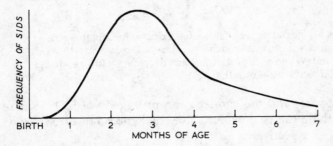

Fig. 4 Age distribution of sudden infant deaths

that at this time SIDS was not only the most common single cause of death, but was greater than all the other causes put together (Fig. 6). This has been one of the ironies of the syndrome – in past years far greater publicity has been given to diseases such as infant leukaemia, cystic fibrosis, spina bifida and others, yet SIDS is much more common than any as a cause of death and *may even be greater than all of them combined* at the peak risk time. Without in any way wishing to diminish the tragedy of these other infant killers or the sterling efforts of parents and doctors to support research into them, it illustrates the fundamental difference between diseases which afflict children more slowly – enabling parents and doctors to get organised and arouse interest and

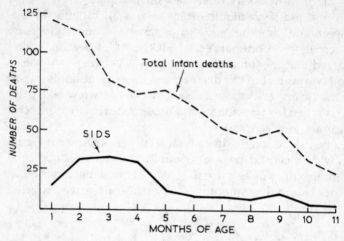

Fig. 5 Age pattern of post-neonatal deaths in Copenhagen, Denmark, both total and due to SIDS, collected over a 10-year period. Whereas the total mortality decreases with age, that of SIDS peaks at 2–4 months

support – and the sudden, abrupt tragedy of SIDS, where nothing can be done for a live child and no research carried out prospectively.

Why SIDS has such a circumscribed age range is still unknown. A number of theories have foundered for lack of proof. One idea was that this was the time when the child's level of immunity was at its lowest ebb. The passive immunity granted from the mother fades after birth and the active resistance to infection generated by the baby itself does not climb to effective levels until well into the first year. However, measurements of the special proteins responsible for immunity failed to show any difference between SIDS victims and control babies. Now that the stability of the breathing mechanism is a major contender for the prime role in SIDS, it is said by some that this is the period during which the maturation of the nervous system controlling breathing is defective – but this does not explain why the younger babies rarely suffer SIDS.

At the present time, all we can say is that we just don't know, but it is certain that something happens in the second half of the first year of life which rapidly takes infants out of the SIDS risk area.

SEX

There is only a slightly greater risk of SIDS in male babies compared to female, this difference being greatest at two months of age. Several surveys have given conflicting results, but most show a slight preponderance of boys. This is of the order of 60:40 per cent boys to girls, but some research has shown there to be no sex difference and two invest-igations actually revealed an excess of girls. However, it may be accepted that the male infant is slightly more at risk,

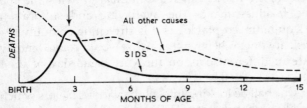

Fig. 6 At about three months, SIDS can equal all other causes

but this is not thought to be related to the basic causes of SIDS. Boys and men are poorer survivors than the so-called 'weaker sex' all through life. Male life expectancy is shorter at all ages and for most diseases and unnatural causes the male invariably comes off worst. The differences in sex incidence in the sudden infant death syndrome show such a small variation that it cannot be significant in any theories of causation.

TWINS

The commonly-quoted figure of 1 in 500 live births for the incidence of SIDS applies only to singletons – that is babies born from a single pregnancy, though of course they may have elder brothers and sisters. Unfortunately, the rate is appreciably higher in twins. One member of a twin pair has a definitely increased susceptibility to cot death, the actual level of increased risk being a matter of some controversy. It was said for a considerable time that the twin had about twice the rate of a single baby in respect of SIDS, but the large investigation in Cardiff covering over 47 000 births between 1965 and 1977 revealed no less than a *five times* increase in the risk of a cot death, from 1.94 to 9.45 per 1000.

On about eight recorded occasions (and undoubtedly many more unrecorded) the overwhelming tragedy of *both* members of a pair of twins dying from SIDS on the same day has been known. Five of these double fatalities came from a survey of 770 cot deaths in Copenhagen, Denmark. Incidentally, all of these babies were found face up in their cots with no bedclothes over the face, but even if this had not been so, the marked increase in SIDS in twins and the multiple fatalities makes the overlaying and suffocation theories quite unacceptable, as it is stretching credulity too far to ask anyone to believe that twins would coincidentally suffocate in different cots on the very same day of their lives.

Later we shall be looking into all the various factors which are thought to contribute to SIDS and it will become apparent that twins suffer more from some of these factors, apart from the uniqueness of being twins. For instance, they are very often premature and are often under normal birth-weight. They more often need to spend the early part of their lives in special care units in maternity hospitals. In most cases twins are bottle fed, though the role of breast feeding in SIDS is a matter of much controversy. All these factors make them more vulnerable to sudden infant death.

The risks of SIDS are the same in both identical and non-identical twins, strongly suggesting that a common environment rather than a genetic factor is responsible. A survey might help to distinguish factors which were hereditary from those which were acquired during the time spent in the common womb and after birth, in a similar environment. In the Copenhagen series mentioned above, the author could not find any similar double fatality in non-twins in the hospitals and children's homes of the city over the previous 50-year period.

SEASONAL FACTORS

Like twins, the time of year has a profound effect on the incidence of sudden infant death. In the northern hemisphere, where most surveys and research have been carried out in Europe and North America, there is an obvious predominance of SIDS in the autumn, winter and spring months – generally from about October until April (Figs. 7, 8 and 9). In Australia the position is reversed and there the

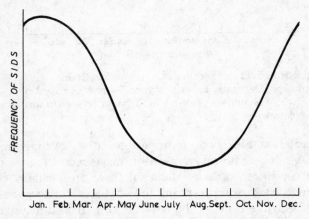

Fig. 7 Seasonal incidence of SIDS in the northern hemisphere

danger period is in the months between March and September because their winter falls in this period. There is obviously a connection between season and weather, rather than a mere calendar effect; later we shall see an equally obvious connection between the frequency of colds and chest infections and the triggering of sudden infant deaths.

Though these autumn, winter and spring months are much more risky for SIDS, cases do occur at all the other times of the year. Figure 8 shows a typical distribution in the northern hemisphere, but there are fatalities in every month, though their comparative rarity is apparent.

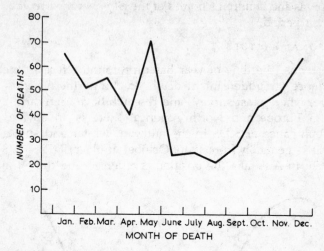

Fig. 8 Seasonal occurrences of sudden infant deaths in Copenhagen, Denmark, in a typical year. There is an excess in winter, with a secondary peak in May; this is often seen in spring in other countries

In addition, SIDS occur in tropical countries, even though we have poorer information about this aspect. In some of these countries, such as Malaysia, there are virtually no different seasons and certainly no cold weather to correspond to winters in the higher latitudes. It is difficult to compare mortality rates for SIDS in many tropical countries or those warmer countries where the temperature swings are less than in the north or south lands. Their high infant mortality rate from other causes, and less efficient registration facilities, hamper any investigation of the relative importance of SIDS. For instance, it would be very difficult indeed to get any idea of the frequency of sudden infant death in rural India, where many *births* go unrecorded, let alone any accurate estimate of infant deaths and the causes of those deaths. The undoubted occurrence of SIDS in virtually all countries, however, makes it apparent that season in itself is not the important factor in terms of climate alone. Almost certainly the prevalence of respiratory infections in the

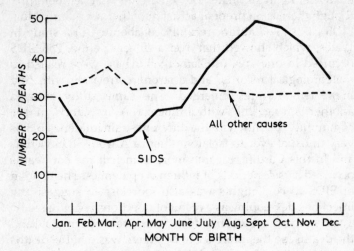

Fig. 9 The months of birth of infants who die between 2–11 months of age in Copenhagen. The SIDS victims show a marked seasonal variation, while 'all other causes' show no change related to time of birth

cooler, damper seasons of temperate climates is an important precipitating factor in SIDS.

Among the very many theories about the syndrome is one which blames temperature directly and it is difficult to decide how much credence to give this view. Almost always it is low temperature that is blamed, though one hypothesis blamed overheating of the infant. A number of investigations have raised some evidence of the involvement of low temperature, though it must immediately be said that this is only likely to be a contributory factor in some of the deaths and certainly can be ruled out in very many tragedies, especially those which occur in hot countries. The author saw SIDS in Malaya, where hypothermia (low temperature) was a physical impossibility! Some of the work pointing a finger at low temperature has come from Canada, where naturally the climatic conditions make hypothermia a real and frequent possibility.

Even in less severe climates, there is some statistical

evidence to incriminate low environmental temperature, though there is no proof of actual hypothermia in individual SIDS cases. The author recently collaborated in a study in Wales, which showed that over a 20-year period, 286 SIDS occurred in one area of Glamorgan. These were related to meteorological records, and a strong correlation with cold night temperatures emerged. The same study showed another strong link with influenza A infections in the community, but not with the different strain influenza B. It is very unusual ever to isolate influenza A from SIDS victims and in this Cardiff research more than half the cot deaths occurred *outside* periods of influenza epidemics. The relation of SIDS to cold nights was also too close to suggest any infections developing as a result of infections encouraged by a cold snap – there was insufficient time between the cold and the deaths, so the inference to be drawn was that the deaths were directly related to the fall in temperature. It seems unlikely that the majority of babies inside houses will be much affected by a drop in the outside temperature, but the possibility of some link exists, though it is by no means accepted generally.

To summarise: the marked seasonal effects are almost certainly due to the increase in colds, coughs and less apparent silent respiratory infections of the upper and lower air-passages which occur in the colder, wetter months. It must be emphasised, as will be discussed later, that this is but one of the components of the multi-factorial situation which is thought to lead to SIDS and not merely an overwhelming infection that directly kills the infant victim.

The timing of SIDS

We have just spoken of the seasonal variations in cot deaths, but there are well-marked variations on a shorter time scale. Sudden infant deaths are more common at week-ends and at holiday times, a fact which is borne out by several surveys, but which is rather hard to explain. Saturday seems the most dangerous day, with Sunday close behind. In the 1974-6 survey in Newcastle-upon-Tyne, 16 of the 29 SIDS occurred at week-ends or bank holidays.

There are, of course, comparable variations in many other kinds of death, in adults and children. Murder, suicide, accidents and even heart attacks vary from one part of the week or month to another – many factors are involved, such as the days on which people get their pay-packet and go drinking, stay in bed later or otherwise alter their usual daily routine. In SIDS, it has been suggested that at the week-ends parents tend to lie-in later and may not look at their infants as often or as early as on other days – the same may apply to public holidays. This sometimes greatly aggravates the feelings of guilt so prevalent in bereaved parents.

As will be mentioned again, SIDS deaths have a strong tendency to occur early in the day. In the Newcastle survey, for instance, 21 of the 29 cases were discovered between 6 a.m. and noon and other investigations in several countries have invariably reported the same finding. Another feature relating to time was also brought out by the Newcastle work, as elsewhere: there tended to be a long interval between the last visit to the baby and the time of discovery of death. In 20 of the 29 SIDS, at least five hours had elapsed since the baby was last looked at by a parent. This is partly explained by the fact that many babies are found dead first thing in the morning, when they naturally may not have been seen since being put to bed the previous evening, but others have been left longer than usual, sometimes due to the more relaxed domestic routine on a week-end or holiday.

Social class variations

This is rather a delicate matter to discuss, as we have to balance the individual infant deaths against the wider epidemiological picture. It is a fairly obvious fact that the type of parent who wants to read this book, who seeks information by writing or phoning the various organisations concerned with SIDS and who in other ways actively seeks counselling, tends to be more vocal and intelligent than the larger proportion of bereaved parents who are never heard from by the organisations and health care people concerned in counselling.

This large, silent majority greatly outnumbers the vocal minority and is known only through the statistical records and the large surveys that have been carried out in Europe, America and Australasia.

From this last source of information it has been found time and time again that there is an undisputable 'social gradient' in the frequency of SIDS, more cases occurring as the social scale is descended. In these egalitarian times, even speaking of social class can be a controversial and delicate matter, but in Britain it is assessed by medical statisticians and the governmental agencies on the basis of the occupation of the head of the household, rather than by trying to classify wealth, educational, racial or other cultural characteristics. The use of the father's occupation is an imperfect method, especially in SIDS, as the man of the family (in some cases) may not be the actual father. A small but significant proportion of mothers may be unmarried or separated.

The method does give a broad measure of the position of the family in the social hierarchy, though anomalies can give rise to obvious fallacies. It sometimes causes offence because no SIDS parent likes to read that the syndrome is much more common in the lower classes, to use an out-dated term.

In Britain this social gradient is measured on the Registrar-General's scale. He is the governmental officer charged with population statistics at the Office of Population Censuses and Surveys, who uses an arbitrary scale for social class descending from Class I through II, III, IV to Class V, depending on the occupation of the husband. Class I consists of professional and upper managerial people; Class II of what might be called middle management, tradespeople and many self-employed; Class III are skilled workers; Class IV semi-skilled persons, and Class V unskilled workers.

This is an almost fatuously simplified description, but gives the general idea, though for the purposes of SIDS investigation, perhaps a classification of the standard of housing might be more accurate. Where a father is unemployed or a serviceman, or where the mother is unmarried, the group is registered as unclassified, which is not very helpful, but unavoidable.

Other methods of estimating social factors rely on residential areas and the standard of housing. They can be seen clearly in relation to SIDS in geographical zones within our cities. Though cot deaths occur everywhere – in the smart commuter belts, the semi-detached suburbs and in country villages – statistically they are concentrated in the city areas of lower social standing. The large council estates of municipal housing and the run-down Victorian terraces of Britain are the centres of SIDS in this country and there are parallels elsewhere, such as crib deaths in the United States. Dr Marie Valdes-Dapena, one of America's leading authorities on SIDS, published an article some years ago containing a map of Philadelphia on which the crib deaths were marked with dots. Beside this was a similar map of the city showing areas which contained dilapidated housing and were scheduled for demolition. The two zones were virtually identical.

In another well-known survey of SIDS, carried out in Newcastle in the mid-1970s, it was found that 45 per cent of all the SIDS in a two-year period occurred in three adjacent city wards which contained only 13 per cent of the infant population. These wards were along the river, consisting of the old run-down industrial areas and among those recognised as stress areas by the local council because they contained a high proportion of households suffering socio-economic deprivation. In the survey, none of the 29 SIDS families owned their own homes and 23 were in council-rented accommodation. Control families in the study showed exactly the opposite trend in living conditions. There were more unemployed fathers in the SIDS families compared with the controls chosen to match the age and sex of the victims. There was not a single parent in the SIDS group who was in social Class I or II.

What does all this mean? There are some very good reasons why SIDS should be more common among the lower social orders, however this is defined. First and most obviously, there are more people in Classes III–V so there is naturally a greater proportion of the population at risk. There are, for instance, far more builders' labourers than there are merchant bankers, and more truck drivers than doctors, so there are bound to be more cot deaths in these groups because there are more families to have more babies.

There are extra factors related to social class. Though not nearly so true now since the advent of widespread family planning, these sections of society tend (or tended) to have larger families than the professional and managerial classes, again causing more babies to be potentially at risk. Their housing is less spacious and more crowded so there is more opportunity for cross-infection for nose, throat and chest infections are undoubtedly a potent factor in at least the triggering of SIDS. There is more chance that one of three children living in the couple of bedrooms of a council house will cough or sneeze his viruses over his infant brother or sister than that the single child in a larger detached house in outer suburbs will catch the same infection.

Other factors, more controversial but sustained by some authorities and surveys, relate socio-economic conditions to standards of mothering care, maternal smoking, feeding habits and even child abuse, but we leave these more sensitive issues until later in our attempts to unravel the complex maternal and family factors, which are sometimes at odds with scientific findings. Suffice it to say that a number of specific risk factors for SIDS have been found to be greater in this section of the community, though it must be emphasised that sudden infant death can – and does – strike at any family, irrespective of the position in the social hierarchy.

Apart from the matters of social class, there are other statistically significant factors which characterise the family in which SIDS tends to occur more often.

The mother is younger, but tends to have several children, compared with control families, which are always an indispensable part of any research investigation. SIDS is less frequent in first-born children; this is one factor (and a weak one) which makes it marginally more likely that a family which has had one SIDS will have a greater risk in subsequent babies, but this slight loading is so tenuous that it is quite legitimate for those counselling SIDS parents to assure them that they have little to fear in the future. The questions always asked by the mother are: 'Is cot death something that runs in the family? Will it happen to my next baby?' The answer is 'almost certainly not'.

Statistically though there is a slightly greater risk in subsequent children of a mother who has already suffered a cot death, the best way to appreciate the tiny added risk is to remember that of the next 500 babies born to parents who have already lost a child from SIDS, 497 will survive and only three will die, contrasted to one death in 500 babies from families who have been free from cot deaths. These odds are great enough for a counsellor to be able to reassure the parents that they have little to fear. The tiny increase in risk already mentioned is because subsequent children will naturally be farther along in the family with the slight loading of risk that this brings. But this is purely a statistical risk and is reduced by the equally inevitable fact that the mother is older by the time another child is born. There is nothing in the baby's constitution that causes this faint increase in risk; it is entirely a maternal factor picked up in statistical analysis but, like so much in the SIDS story, remains unexplained.

Sometimes reports of multiple SIDS appear in the Press, often over-sensationalised and inaccurate, as unfortunately so much tends to be in the popular media about SIDS. Though on purely mathematical grounds the tragedy of a second cot death in the same family is bound to happen now and again (perhaps about three times a year in Britain), a third death is bound to be incredibly rare. Yet reports are made of three, four or even five infant deaths in a family and the blame is laid at the door of the sudden infant death syndrome. This is virtually impossible and some other disease process must be involved. There are several rare inborn metabolic diseases, often hereditary, which can cause multiple deaths in a family. These diseases affect the chemistry of the body and may be difficult to detect, but they must certainly be the explanation for these excessively rare, but over-publicised tragedies.

In the Newcastle series, which is representative of many such investigations in different parts of the world, there was a significant excess of mothers under 21 years of age and of fathers under 25. Other family factors, which will be explored in more detail, include the amount of breast feeding, the proportion of mothers who smoked and, very importantly, the irregularity of attendance at ante-natal and child clinics.

PREMATURITY

There is no doubt that the risk of a sudden death is increased in babies born before the full forty-week duration of pregnancy. This also applies to babies significantly under the average normal birth-weight, whether they were premature or not, though naturally the two conditions very often occur together. The marked increase in the incidence of SIDS in babies who had been admitted to neonatal intensive care units is largely related to prematurity and low birth-weight, because these are the infants who need such strenuous care to help them retain their fragile hold on life. Recent theorising leads us to believe that prematurity causes not only the body size to be small, but that control mechanisms in brain and perhaps heart may also be immature for a number of months after birth, leading to breathing and circulatory instability related to the causes of cot death.

ILLEGITIMACY

This has also been statistically shown to lead to a higher SIDS rate. Obviously this can be due only to secondary associations, such as a more frequent lower position in the Registrar-General's scale, often poorer housing accommodation and perhaps a reduced willingness to take advantage of ante-natal and post-natal care.

SMOKING HABITS OF THE MOTHER

Quite a strong association of smoking with SIDS has been shown, though again it is difficult to know whether this is a direct link or merely an association with social factors. In the Cardiff survey of almost 50 000 births, it was found that the rate of sudden infant death in non-smoking or ex-smoking mothers was 1.18 per 1000 live births. If the mother smoked less than 20 cigarettes a day, the risk rose to 2.6 per 1000 but if she smoked more than 20 a day, it jumped to 5.62, over five times that of non-smokers.

ATTENDANCE AT ANTE-NATAL CLINIC

Several surveys have shown that the SIDS rate is related to the enthusiasm with which a mother goes to clinic during pregnancy. This is so firmly related that it has been used as one of the predictive factors to detect high-risk babies in surveys to be described later. In the Cardiff survey, published in 1982, the over-all rate of sudden infant death during the 12 years studied was 2.1 per 1000 live births. Where the mother attended 15 or more clinic sessions, the rate dropped to only 0.73, but where she went only three or four times, it rose to 3.38 and where the mothers attended less than three times, it jumped to 6.34.

As was shown in the famous Sheffield survey, it is the whole picture of general maternal care and standard of mothering that seems related to the SIDS rate rather than any specific medical intervention ... and this is in turn statistically linked to social class factors as well as to geography and housing standards.

THE ROLE OF BREAST FEEDING IN SIDS

A very common query comes both from parents and from medical and paramedical people, when discussing sudden infant death. 'Does breast feeding prevent cot death?' they ask. The answer is rather hard to give as either 'yes or no'. There is no doubt that, statistically, SIDS is less common among mothers who breast feed their babies, but the reasons are not as simple as that fact would suggest. The problem is partly that of parallel associations, in that in a society such as Western Europe and similar communities in North America and Australasia, the prevalence of breast feeding may be related to social class differences and to standards of mothering. The author hastily adds that exceptions are legion, but we are talking about statistics. In the widest sense, the keen mother who is determined to breast feed is often the one who faithfully attends every clinic and who might be more alert to detecting early signs of even minor illness in the baby. In several SIDS surveys, such as that of Professor Emery in Sheffield, attendance at clinic and the fact and even intention of breast feeding, were all advantageous factors when assessing prospective risks of a cot death.

Therefore it cannot be said from these facts that it is some physical property of breast milk itself that protects against SIDS, but rather parallel factors perhaps more related to the maternal and social situation.

For many other medical and obstetrical reasons, there is absolutely no doubt that breast feeding is to be highly recommended, from psychological aspects for both mother and baby and for the optimum nutritional value – cow's milk was meant for calves, not humans! In addition, mother's milk contains anti-infection elements that must help towards a healthier baby, though not necessarily in relation to sudden infant death. It is therefore difficult to evaluate the contribution of breast feeding in this context; there is no doubt whatsoever that many SIDS occur in wholly breast-fed babies, both today and especially in former years. Bottle feeding is a relatively new phenomenon and down the centuries – and in less sophisticated communities today – the vast majority of babies have fed and still feed at the breast, often until a far greater age than most modern, westernised infants.

No doubt the mother in Solomon's case 3000 years ago was breast fed, yet SIDS occur in all lands and in all times. That SIDS quite often occurs in totally breast-fed infants is beyond dispute; at the 1974 Seattle meeting, Dr Abraham Bergman, one of the most experienced SIDS workers in the United States, stated categorically that he knew of 50 or 60 families, who totally employed breast feeding for their infants, yet suffered a crib death. All other doctors concerned with SIDS have similar experiences. He went on to say, 'Our feeling is that it is wrong to impugn guilt in literature that is supposed to help people, while the question remains without a scientific answer. I happen to believe in breast feeding and I think it is better for a whole lot of reasons; but I don't think that people who have lost crib death babies should have it suggested to them that their baby might still be alive if they had only breast fed.'

This then is the situation – it is better to breast-feed, especially during the period immediately after the birth, but although there is some statistical evidence that SIDS deaths occur somewhat less often in those families who breast-feed, there is no direct evidence that it is the actual milk that makes the difference. Another aspect, of course, is that until a very few years ago breast feeding was unpopular in modern society and the statistical comparisons of a small minority of breast-feeders with the huge majority of bottle-fed babies made the significance less sure. In addition, many allegedly breast-fed babies were often put on a bottle, either as a supplement when breast-milk was scanty or as an occasional convenience. When the interest in cow's-milk allergy as a cause of cot death was popular, it was found that even a couple of bottles of cow's milk given at intervals in an otherwise breast-fed baby, was quite effective in producing antibodies to cow's-milk protein in the baby's blood. It was quite hard at that time to find many babies who were genuinely *totally* breast-fed, but breastfeeding has regained much popularity in very recent times, partly as a result of the exhortations of doctors and from the increase in women's desire to return to more natural ways of living, feeding and giving birth.

To summarise, though there is no direct evidence that breast feeding protects against SIDS: the medical student's old proverb recommending breast-milk can be safely adopted … 'It's free, it's nutritious, it's sterile, it's warm – and it comes in such attractive containers!'

2 · The typical tragedy –
an all too familiar story

We have looked at the over-all pattern of babes at risk, though we must come back to look at it in more depth later. The individual tragedy itself must now be described, a poignant but necessary story which contrasts with the impersonal approach of statistics and epidemiology.

The first thing to notice is the remarkable uniformity of most instances of SIDS. When a pathologist is requested by the coroner to perform a post-mortem examination, he usually gets a brief preliminary history of the circumstances from the coroner's officer, either on a history sheet or dictated over the telephone. So constant and repetitive are most of the cot death histories that a rubber stamp could be made to record them rather than the effort of writing out each one.

The mother tells how she put her baby to sleep at night, the infant being either in perfectly good health or with trivial symptoms, and finds it dead in the cot in the morning. This simple but devastating story is repeated many hundreds of times each year in Britain and thousands of times in the United States, with or without slight variations.

As mentioned, the baby was thought to be perfectly well in at least half the cases; the mother will have noticed nothing wrong with it during the preceding day or usually during the previous few days. Some scientific evidence has been found in recent years to suggest that some of these 'well' babes were in fact not so well internally, but using symptoms and appearances as the best maternal guide, the fact remains that almost as many infants seemed in good health as those that had some recorded ailment. Closer examination may, however, alter superficial impressions. The other half of the cases were said to have had something amiss – usually quite trivial and not sufficient in the majority of instances to cause the mother any concern nor to lead her to call the doctor. Most often these symptoms were merely a cold or a snuffly nose or perhaps loose bowel motions. The babe might have been slightly off colour in a vague way, the mother thinking that though it had nothing specifically wrong, it was just not as bright as usual.

Even these reports on about half the infant victims said to have had slight symptoms must be examined rather critically. Remember that the history was taken almost immediately after a shattering and bewildering tragedy, the worst thing by far ever to have happened, or likely to happen, to the poor mother. She, desperately trying to rationalise the fact of her baby's death, dredges up every tiny fact and recent happening to try and explain the death to herself, even more than to the interviewer. The snuffles and the cold, the loose motion – all these have to be evaluated in the context of babies in autumn, winter and spring, when a significant proportion of the infant population have snuffles, colds or a little diarrhoea.

Even when allowance is made for the over-emphasis produced by the desperate searching of the mother's memory when giving her story, there seems to be no doubt that a significant number of SIDS victims have had some mild symptoms – usually of a respiratory infection – in the few days before the death. In the Newcastle-upon-Tyne series, for example, of the 29 deaths, 9 had significant symptoms, 12 had trivial complaints and 8 had none whatsoever. These findings, inevitably recorded in retrospect, are perhaps a little stronger than many other series. The standards set by different investigators causes some variation. For example, Professor John Emery, the Sheffield doyen of British SIDS investigation, draws a much more serious picture of pre-tragedy symptoms than has been formerly accepted by most investigators of the cot death syndrome – and what John Emery says needs to be taken very seriously. According to data from Sheffield published in 1979, symptoms were much more common than thought previously and the number of symptoms in a given child were related to the actual risk of a SIDS taking place. In all 97 sudden unexpected infant deaths were investigated and compared with control babies born at almost the same time. It was found that in the three weeks prior to death the 97 SIDS had 260 recorded symptoms between them, but the controls only had 48 symptoms. Only 7 of the SIDS were said to be absolutely symptom-free, but the 64 of the controls had no symptoms. A total of 84 per cent of the SIDS had more than one symptom, but only 30 per cent of the controls had multiple signs. There were 31 different symptoms recorded, but the 9 most common were snuffles, cough, irritability, vomiting, diarrhoea, drowsiness, a rash, change of cry and a temperature. Of all these, snuffles was the most common.

The next modification of the standard history is that the child may not have been found dead in its sleeping place first thing in the morning, but a little later. For example, a common story is of the mother–or, indeed, the father – looking at the baby or perhaps giving it its early morning feed at around six o'clock. Then the mother goes back to bed, or the father goes off to work, and the child is left to sleep on until breakfast time. As mentioned earlier, a number of the week-end deaths may be discovered later in the morning, after the parents have had a lie-in. In any event, the child is revisited later and the parent is devastated to find it still and lifeless in its cot.

The most common story is to hear of the infant's being found dead in the early part of the day and, as mentioned in the previous chapter, several surveys as well as general medical experience have shown that death occurs before ten o'clock in the morning in most tragedies and that at least 60 per cent take place before noon. Fewer occur at other times of the day, and SIDS rarely occur in the evening–though if no other explanation is forthcoming after all the investigations have been completed and if the rest of the circumstances fit, then, by exclusion, these few cases have to be categorised as sudden infant death syndrome.

The very description cot or crib death indicates that the children die in their sleeping place, while asleep. This is very relevant to current theories of the cause of SIDS, which is examined in a later chapter. In the Newcastle series of 29 SIDS, 8 infants died in their cots, 10 in perambulators (where many babies habitually sleep all night), 7 in carry-cots and the remaining 4 in the parental bed.

The circumstances of the discovery of the death vary considerably. The shock and its consequences experienced by the mother will be dealt with later, but here we are concerned with the actual event. In most instances, the babe is found lying face up, with the bedclothes, blankets and covers well away from the face, so that there is no possibility whatsoever of suffocation. In a substantial number, however, the child may be in a posture which gives credence to the old arguments about asphyxia—though this is quite illogical as no one disputes that most infants die in a position where this could not happen. So how can the suffocation advocates summon any proof for their theories when far more babies die in conditions which exclude suffocation? And how can the suffocation advocates fit their theory into the well-known pattern of increased risk in a twin, the marked social class variation, the slight sex variation, the seasonal differences and all the other unrelated factors that will come to light in later discussion?

This is by no means an academic argument, as will be made clear later on, but it is essential to defeat the remarkably persistent rumour that mechanical suffocation has anything to do with SIDS. The author once went to great lengths in a television interview to explain how natural disease and not suffocation was the cause of cot deaths—but the programme presenters followed his item immediately with a demonstration by a highly uninformed health visitor of how the bedclothes in a cot caused babies to asphyxiate! Things are better these days, but the old legend dies hard.

The babies who are found not face up and uncovered may be found buried under a heap of blankets, which is a fairly common way for some babies to sleep—the vast majority of whom thankfully never suffer a cot death. They may even be found huddled up in a corner of the cot with a mound of clothes over them in what appears to be a very unnatural and uncomfortable position ... but for every SIDS baby found like that, there will be thousands of healthy children cramped into the same position. It's just one way in which some babies sleep. There may be one or more blankets over the face of a SIDS victim or over a legion of normally healthy, surviving infants and this fact is irrelevant in the context of the cause of SIDS.

Many other babies, of course, sleep face down, either half on one side or often flat on their stomachs, face in the pillow. Unfortunately—and quite understandably when cot death has been such a mystery for centuries – this has been so often suggested and accepted as the reason for the death. The apparent blockage of the nose and mouth by the pillow – or the mattress if the baby slips down into the bed – may be thought to have caused suffocation, but as so many healthy babies sleep like this, it is patently untrue.

Years ago it was found that all fabrics used in the manufacture of bed coverings, such as woollen blankets, cotton and nylon sheets and other man-made fabrics, easily admitted enough air through the weave to allow full respiration for the relatively slight needs of an infant. Naturally, impervious membranes such as rubber or polythene cannot admit air, but these are never used as top coverings or as the uppermost layer underneath a child. Unless the baby is ill and inert, it will not get into a position where the weight of its head can press the nose and mouth into an impervious substance. Other tests – and the experience of countless mothers, nurses and doctors – have proved that a baby will lift and turn its head away from such obstructions in a search for air.

Later on, we shall look at the possibility that partial blockage of the internal air passages by disease or slow development may play a contributory role in SIDS, but present insistence on the lack of proof that external suffocation is the cause of cot deaths is due to the great psychological danger to the mother of accepting such an unlikely theory.

The awful moment – and after

The reactions of the person who discovers the infant vary considerably, but it would seem that a paralysing disbelief is more common than a violent or hysterical outburst. Grief tends to develop gradually and will be discussed at length later in the book. Not uncommonly, the complete opposite of disbelief occurs.

Mothers have described how they were immediately aware that their baby was dead. Naturally, the mother most often discovers the tragedy and, from the hundreds of letters and conversations describing the moment, it seems that in many instances the mother instinctively knows that her child has passed away, even before she picks it up. Some mothers recall a desperate, icy calm, as if the event is not really happening or is some nightmare from which she will soon awake. These are natural defensive reactions, an effort to shut out the truth by temporarily denying that it has actually happened.

In perhaps the majority of cases, however, the mother is suddenly appalled to find that something is dreadfully amiss with her baby, though at that moment the possibility of its death does not enter her mind, being too cruel a thought to be contemplated. She may see that the child is still, apparently not breathing and is either ashen pale in colour or slightly blue, especially about the lips. Her instinctive reaction is to snatch up the child and rush off to get help, either from a neighbour, the family doctor or a hospital. Other mothers will dash off for help without the child, seeking aid from someone in the house, or a neighbour, or from the first passer-by in the street.

In towns and cities, the mother quite often phones the ambulance service and these experienced men may be on the scene within minutes, offering artificial respiration and oxygen. Occasionally, their efforts are rewarded and the saved child then becomes a near-miss cot death, a group which will be described in the chapter on theories of the causes of SIDS. In other cases, the family doctor may arrive though often he cannot be found immediately, being either on house visits or at surgery.

Frequently it is obvious to the mother, the family and perhaps the ambulance crew that the baby has gone beyond any hope of revival and there has to be an official pronouncement of death. Unless the family doctor comes to the house quickly, this is usually done at the accident or emergency department of the local hospital, where the child is taken. The problems associated with this first contact with a hospital will be developed later on, but at some point a doctor will have to confirm that the baby is dead. It is here that sometimes the system begins to break down. Many reports from parents have shown that, however unwittingly, the rather stereotyped routines of hospital procedure tend to alienate the parents, especially when they abruptly separate the dead infant from the mother at the time of the confirmation of death.

The legal processes begin

In England and Wales – and in most other countries where there is a set procedure for investigating all deaths that have not occurred under medical care – a SIDS death will have to be reported to a coroner or the equivalent legal authority. Here we must explain the significance of this formality because it has often caused added stress to the family and been felt as some stigma. This in turn has led to a reinforcement of the feelings of self-reproach and guilt universally felt by the mother and has on occasions also led to unjustified criticism by neighbours and even relatives.

In England and Wales about two-thirds of all deaths are dealt with solely by the medical attendant, either the family doctor where the death occurs at home, or a clinician in hospital.

The doctor can complete a death certificate without reference to the coroner if:

(a) he is the regular medical attendant of the deceased

(b) he has seen the patient during life at some time within the fourteen days immediately previous to the death or

(c) has examined the body after death (an unsatisfactory alternative as he should always do this in any case)

(d) he is satisfied as to the medical cause of death

(e) he is entirely satisfied that the death was due to natural disease.

If he can satisfy all these criteria then the doctor completes a medical certificate of the cause of death, which is either sent or taken by relatives to the local registrar of births and deaths, who issues a disposal order which allows burial (though not cremation, for which further certificates have to be obtained).

If these criteria cannot be satisfied, then the doctor – if there is one – should report the case to the coroner immediately. In some instances, the report will be made by the registrar, usually because the doctor's certificate does not fulfill all the criteria mentioned above.

THE CORONER

The coroner is a lawyer (and, in a few places such as London, also a doctor) charged with the investigation of all deaths reported to him, that is those not covered by the usual medical certificate of death. About 30 per cent of all deaths in England and Wales are reported to the coroner, the vast majority being cases in which the medical attendant has not seen the deceased within the last fortnight before death and therefore cannot issue a certificate.

The office of coroner is one of the most ancient in English legal history, dating back to at least the twelfth century. Though the coroner was originally most concerned with the administration of justice, especially the collection of fines, in the last couple of centuries his major role has been to detect unnatural deaths, especially those which may have been due to concealed criminal activity. In the past few decades, this role has changed again in some measure. The vast majority of cases are screened for other reasons: unexpected natural death, accidents, suicides, industrial diseases and other matters where, although there may be an unnatural element in the death, it is rarely criminal. In fact, the investigation of potentially criminal deaths is now carried out almost entirely by the Criminal Investigation Department (CID) police forces and sent to Crown Courts. The coroner has lost most of his jurisdiction in criminal matters, except for a formal inquest where no culprit has been detected. Unfortunately, this former major role of the coroner, which was so strong in the last century, is still felt to be a social stigma by many people who do not understand the evolution of his procedure. In fact, since some recent legislation during the past five years, the coroner has lost virtually all his criminal jurisdiction, being unable to send persons for trial from his inquests and even forbidden to impute criminal actions or even negligence to any person.

All this is very relevant in the context of cot death. In former years—and possibly in a few outposts today—coroners were the cause for increasing parental suffering by injudicious comments and attitudes, usually during public inquests. The ever-present feelings of guilt suffered by the mother of a recent cot death can be greatly reinforced by unnecessary repetition in a coroner's court and by criticism from a coroner, who often has no medical qualifications. Thankfully this aspect of the problem has all but vanished, but some facets of the legal procedure still cause unnecessary suffering and will be discussed later.

In countries other than England and Wales, either a modified coroner's system or a different procedure is followed. For instance, in Scotland there is no coroner, but the procurator fiscal occupies a broadly similar function. In the United States, either coroners or Medical Examiners provide the legal machinery for the investigation of sudden deaths and again there can be great variation in practice from one place to another. In many countries which were formerly part of the British Empire, the coroner's system persists, such as Canada, Australia and New Zealand. In other areas such as the continent of Europe, a different system more directly associated with judicial enquiries is in existence. However, in most of these countries, where there is a well-organised legal system, all deaths which cannot be certified as natural causes by a physician are referred for some kind of medico-legal enquiry.

Going back to our main theme and using England and Wales as an example of the procedure, we find that the individual cot death by definition must be reported to the coroner for medico-legal investigation. Though it is possible – and occasionally done – that such a case might be certified in the usual manner without reporting to the coroner, this would be very exceptional. The reasons are obvious – the infant may not have been seen by the doctor within the previous fortnight because in the vast majority of cases the baby was either quite well or had only trivial symptoms, not necessitating the attention of the family practitioner. Although some cases may have been seen by the doctor, either because the parents called him or took the child to the clinic, circumstances will almost invariably have caused the doctor to withhold a death certificate and inform the coroner.

The deaths are certainly sudden and certainly unexpected and even if the doctor had seen the baby recently, these two facts would have led him to report the case. A most potent factor in any case is the doctor's inability to give a cause of death, which he could naturally not anticipate in a child he either had not seen or may have seen only for trivial symptoms. All these factors combine to make the reporting of the death to the coroner virtually inevitable. Again, a considerable proportion of SIDS are rushed to a hospital casualty department and there the hospital doctor has naturally never had any contact with the family before. He is therefore not the 'regular medical attendant' and is totally unable to certify the cause of death of a child brought to him after any hope of resuscitation has passed.

Reporting a case to the coroner usually means telephoning the coroner's officer, who is often a plain-clothes police officer who acts as the administrative assistant to the coroner and is the contact and liaison between the public and the investigation. This is usually the situation in cities and towns of any size, but in rural areas there may be no coroner's officer. The first police constable involved in the case acts as the coroner's officer for that one death. This again has particular relevance for SIDS as the regular coroner's officer is usually a mature and experienced man, doing nothing else but dealing with sudden deaths and bereaved relatives all day and every day. Where a local police constable is involved, however, it may be the first SIDS case he has ever seen – or ever heard of – and in some instances might be the very first sudden death of any kind which has come his way. In these cases, the administrative pathway may not be very smooth and there are other problems associated with SIDS, which may also appear even where there is a regular coroner's officer and which will be discussed later (see p. 121).

Once he has reported to the coroner, the family doctor's (or hospital clinician's) legal responsibility ceases and, regrettably, it sometimes ceases in all other respects so that the relatives get very little support from the medical person involved. Once the coroner is informed of the death, it is entirely up to him to decide what shall be done about it in the way of investigation. In the vast majority of cases – and in cot death almost invariably – he will order a post-mortem examination to be carried out by a pathologist. This is virtually inevitable because without such an examination no cause of death can be decided and no conclusion reached which can be certified as the cause on the eventual death certificate.

Even though the syndrome of cot death is now very well recognised – compared to the situation 20 years ago – the sudden, unexpected mode of death in itself means that a post-mortem examination (often called an 'autopsy' or 'necropsy') is the only sure means of distinguishing the true SIDS from other diseases or sometimes even unnatural causes which may be present. Though the autopsy findings in SIDS are essentially negative, this exclusion of other causes together with the typical history is sufficient to categorise the death for statistical and epidemiological research purposes and to satisfy the legal processes that no criminal or accidental action is being concealed. The negative result may not be much help to the parents waiting anxiously for some answer to their questions, but with adequate explanation by a doctor or other health care worker, the negative findings can be put into the right context in a relatively satisfactory way.

THE POST-MORTEM EXAMINATION

Quite naturally, many parents are very upset by the prospect of a post-mortem examination being held upon their child, an ordeal which may seem a cruel and unnecessary additional burden to the grief which sudden bereavement has brought them. However, most parents accept, albeit reluctantly, that this is the only sensible course, which will at least give them some answers, some reasons. Most parents have an intense need to know why the child was taken from them so abruptly and the uncertainty of no true cause of death being given is one of the most unsatisfactory aspects of the formalities following the death.

The coroner—or his equivalent in other countries—will request an experienced pathologist to conduct the examination, which is usually carried out quite soon after the death, in most cases later that day or on the following day. The pathologist will usually be either a forensic pathologist in a larger city with a medical school—a forensic pathologist being a pathologist who deals exclusively with the legal aspect of pathology—or a hospital pathologist in those areas without a medical school.

The object of the post-mortem examination is three-fold: First to ascertain the medical cause of death; second to exclude any unnatural cause; and last to collect information which, both statistically and by direct investigation, aids in the now widespread research into the causes of cot death which is the only hope for prevention in the future.

The results of the post-mortem examination are complex and may vary in nature from one pathologist to another and from one medical centre to another, depending on the opinions and training of the pathologist involved. Any variations tend to be rather academic in nature, however, and will be discussed further in the chapter on medical theories of the cause of SIDS. In former years – though there are still a few pockets of less satisfactory opinion – some of the very variable and often unsubstantiated opinions of pathologists led to further confusion and sometimes distress for the relatives. At the present time, the most likely source of distress in respect of the post-mortem examination and the pathologist is lack of communication, rather than dubious information. It is still unfortunately the case that in some areas, the parents are not fully informed of the results of the post-mortem examination and may know the actual cause of death only after an undesirable delay. Fortunately it is now becoming a much more widespread practice for the pathologist to meet the parents and explain in non-medical language the findings and the nature of SIDS or, if the pathologist himself does not wish to do this, a paediatrician may take on the same informative role.

The post-mortem examination itself usually takes about an hour or so to perform and the result will be notified to the coroner's officer within a very short time, usually by telephone, followed within a day or two by a written report.

The actual findings are usually so scanty as to have been one of the reasons why SIDS has remained an obscure condition for so long. The post-mortem appearances also have unfortunately helped to reinforce the erroneous assumptions about an asphyxial cause, which has in turn led to many harmful misapprehensions about suffocation.

On examination, the infant victims of SIDS are usually found to be well nourished and without any external indication of disease. A slight discolouration of the lips and ears is not specific of any particular condition, neither is the presence of vomit or stomach contents at the lips or nostrils, as this can occur as a result of the dying process or even after death. Sometimes a little frothy fluid, occasionally pink-stained, may be present at the nostrils or mouth. Again this is from waterlogging of the lungs which occurs in the last moments of life and is not a specific sign which assists in determining the cause of death.

Some parents–and indeed doctors–may be concerned about so-called 'pressure marks' on the face. As many babies sleep either partly or fully on their face, they may die in this position merely because that was the posture when the SIDS struck them. In these cases, especially if the child has not been discovered for some time after death, there may be a white mark covering the nose and mouth which is very evident because the surrounding skin of the face may be pink or bluish in colour, the contrast making the pale area all the more prominent. This sign has been misinterpreted in the past as evidence of suffocation because the baby lay face down on a pillow and therefore was deprived of air. This is not a tenable theory and such appearances are post-mortem in nature due to the settling of the blood in the other parts of the face but not in the area which has been pressed against the pillow by the dead weight of the head.

It is rare among external signs for any obvious indication of illness to be discovered, such as signs of dehydration. In some babies who die of other specific causes over a period of a day or so, there may be loss of body water which causes the skin to be wrinkled and lax: in addition, the fontanelle (space between the skull bones which can be felt on the upper part of the front of the scalp) may be sunken due to the loss of fluid within. In SIDS, though some cases may show biochemical signs of dehydration, these anatomical features are very unusual.

Internally, there is very little to be seen with the naked eye in a typical sudden infant death syndrome. Of babies who die suddenly and unexpectedly in their sleeping places, and which may be classed as cot deaths, about 85 per cent reveal no naked-eye pathological disease to account for death. In these, the cause of death is then attributed to the sudden infant death syndrome, so that they are both cot deaths and SIDS.

The remaining 15 per cent (which in some pathologists' series is considerably more) post-mortem examination reveals some obvious abnormality, which is usually given as the actual cause of death. Therefore, though these are cot deaths in the general sense they are not necessarily SIDS. However, it must be said that a proportion of this 15 per cent, where something definite is found, is still actually SIDS, because although there may be some obvious disease process present, it need not necessarily be the condition which caused death, which still may be the sudden infant death syndrome. For instance, a child may have a congenital defect in the heart which normally may be endured quite tolerably until late in life, but if this is found in a cot death it is usually given as the cause of death. Similarly, a child might have Down's syndrome (mongolism) and may be found suddenly and unexpectedly dead. Again there is a tendency to use the Down's syndrome as the cause of death though in fact it is really a SIDS case in a Down's baby.

Obviously there is a proportion where genuine natural disease was the cause of death: these cases are sometimes frank chest infections, such as a broncho-pneumonia or, in the young infants at the lower end of cot death age range, a brain membrane haemorrhage, usually a sequel to a difficult delivery. It must be emphasised that these cases are comparatively rare and that the vast majority of children in this age group who are found suddenly and unexpectedly dead in their cots are the true SIDS. This is based upon the naked-eye examination by the pathologist: when microscopic examination is conducted, then there is a wider field for a professional difference of opinion in some of the cases, which will be discussed later.

In the typical SIDS, the only constant pathological finding, which is so non-specific as not to give any clue as to the mechanism of the syndrome, is a congestion and often waterlogging of the lungs with some patchy collapse of the periphery of the lungs. In addition, there are usually a number of small to moderate-sized haemorrhages, usually about the size of the head of a pin, scattered on the surface of the lungs, on the surface of the heart and in the large thymus gland which occupies the upper part of the chest.

Unfortunately, these so-called 'serous' haemorrhages or 'petechiae', have long been associated with mechanical asphyxia, such as may be seen in manual strangulation and suffocation. In recent years it has been shown that this association is by no means invariable, such serious haemorrhages being found in all types of death when subjected to post-mortem examination. In addition, true suffocation in infants, which occasionally occurs, may show no such haemorrhages. Thus these petechial haemorrhages are completely non-specific and there is now good evidence to suggest that some of them may be actually post-mortem phenomena. In any case, it is now considered that they arise as an 'agonal' process, being due to rupture of tiny blood vessels under the unsupported membranes of the lung and heart, in the final moments of life when a rise in the pressure in the veins and lack of oxygen in the blood lead to these pin-point bleeding spots. Some authorities in SIDS research maintain that they are due to efforts to breathe against a closed air passage, either a closed larynx (voice box) or the back of the nose and throat. In the present state of knowledge, this is not certain, but what is certain is that these are not signs of mechanical asphyxia from suffocation. This digression into pathology is very relevant, because, as it has been stated several times before, the feelings of recrimination on the part of the parents, especially the mother, are greatly reinforced by any medical comment or opinion which suggests that some form of suffocation led to the death. This was formerly particularly relevant in the so-called over-laying, which will be referred to later: when this explanation fell from favour, the alternative culprits of suffocation such as soft pillows and heavy bedclothes were called in to explain the petechial haemorrhages, but it is now known that no such explanation is necessary.

The other possible finding of the pathologist in SIDS is the presence of some form of respiratory infection, which as we shall see is an important contribution to the triggering of the syndrome. Most post-mortem examinations reveal no genuine respiratory infection, either in the throat, air passages or lungs. However, a relatively small proportion may show a slight reddening of either the interior of the larynx or the windpipe. The lungs never show frank broncho-pneumonia in a case which is considered to be a SIDS rather than a definite chest infection, but the presence of waterlogging and patchy collapse is so common in the SIDS lungs that some pathologists are suspicious that some very early or mild infective change might be present. As will be seen later, this may influence them in their choice of terminology when giving the cause of death.

Because SIDS is such an obscure pathological condition – a challenge to every pathologist – the naked-eye appearances are always followed by a microscopic examination of parts of the various organs, especially the lungs. This takes time and it is usually a minimum of a few days before such tissues are processed by the laboratory and made available for the pathologist to study. Because of this delay, many pathologists will issue their cause of death on the naked-eye findings, this action being made in the light of past experience, which indicates that microscopic examination may not add much to the findings at the original post-mortem. Another reason for issuing a cause of death soon after the post-mortem examination, before the microscopic details are known, is that the coroner wishes to expedite the disposal of the case and the parents naturally wish to know the cause of death and to make their funeral arrangements with a minimum of delay. Nevertheless, some pathologists will delay giving their cause of death until the microscopic examination is made. This practice has much to commend it in scientific terms, as occasionally the naked-eye diagnosis may have to be changed, a difficult if not impossible process once the first opinion as to the cause of death has been registered.

Microscopic examination may reveal better evidence of an early chest infection than was suspected from the naked-eye examination or may confirm the suspicions of the patholo-gist, but this is the exception rather than the rule and is a point about which some pathologists have differences of opinion. The examination of the lungs of an infant by microscopic means is difficult to interpret: experienced paediatric pathologists (those who deal exclusively with childhood diseases) tend to attach more significance to minimal findings than do general and forensic pathologists who deal largely with adult cases. The subject will be explored more deeply in the chapter on the medical research aspects (p. 66), but suffice it to say here that medical opinion is not unanimous on what really constitutes a genuine respiratory infection. The diagnosis is usually made on the presence or absence of inflammatory cells scattered along the air passages and in the lungs. When these are very few in number it becomes a matter of pathological opinion as to whether they constitute evidence of an infection or not. Another problem is that the infection most likely to be involved is due to a virus, in which case the accumulation of inflammatory cells is often slight and delayed. It may well be that a severe virus infection may be present, death occurring before the characteristic accumulation of inflammatory cells has had time to take place.

This again has practical relevance for the parents because the cause of death may be modified by the opinion and past experience of the pathologist.

THE CAUSE OF DEATH

In Solomon's time, it would appear that cot death was called overlaying and this practice has gone on through the centuries until the present time, as there are one or two doctors who consider that it still might be the cause of some cot deaths. The term 'overlaying' tended to vanish, however, about the time of the Second World War. Throughout the ages until the first quarter of this century, it was very common for young babies to sleep in the family bed, except in the upper strata of society. The beds were often deep and soft with feather mattresses and mothers were then not so figure-conscious as now so that they might be of more ample proportions. When a cot death occurred and the infant was found dead in the maternal bed in the morning, it was very natural for everyone to assume that the unfortunate baby had been suffocated by being buried in the deep mattress by the pressure of an adult body.

Indeed, there is still a law in Britain (the Children and Young Persons Act) which categorically states that an adult is guilty of a criminal offence if he or she goes to bed in a drunken condition with an infant which is later found dead. This is probably an example of legislation passed to protect against a condition which does not exist!

With social changes and an increase in the standard of living, most infants were given a separate sleeping place during the past half century or so and therefore overlaying, by definition, could not take place as it is impossible to overlay a child in a cot physically separated from the adult bed. But sudden infant deaths went on occurring just as before. Obviously the overlaying theory was vanquished, but because there was no alternative satisfactory medical explanation for the deaths, the protagonists of suffocation from overlaying merely moved their theorising to other forms of asphyxia. They alleged that the babies died because they were face down in soft pillows, because their faces were covered by heavy bedclothes or even that they had been suffocated by cats sleeping upon the face! The presence of the pin-point haemorrhages on the lungs continued to support this unprovable theory. However, various workers in the medical field showed that bedclothes were quite pervious to air in the quantities needed for infant breathing, that a previously healthy child would always turn its head away from a suffocating pillow and that the likelihood of cats sleeping upon 2000 infants and causing their death each year in Britain, was highly unlikely. In addition, it was well recognised that many SIDS died on their backs with their faces clear of the bedclothes.

At the beginning of the Second World War, the pathology services in Britain were greatly improved, especially by the establishment of the Emergency Medical Service Hospitals with their increasingly numerous pathology staffs. These pathologists performed more and more post-mortem examinations for coroners and became very conscious that the old theories of suffocation were unacceptable in the cot death cases with which they had to deal.

The pathologists were faced with a dilemma – they wished to avoid using inaccurate and harmful terms like suffocation and overlaying because these inevitably led to the presumption that the death was unnatural and therefore an inquest had to be held with all the attendant troubles for the parents. The pathologists became convinced that the deaths were due to natural causes but were completely unsure as to the nature of the natural disease. If they were completely honest, they would have to write 'unascertainable' or 'unknown' as the cause of death, but this in itself would lead to exactly the same situation as using the term suffocation in that there would have to be an inquest.

To avoid this situation, the practice grew of calling the death the result of a respiratory infection. In some cases the pathologist did not really believe this, so it was a legal fiction or white lie for the benefit of the parents. The coroner usually knew this and went along with the mild deception in order to assist the feelings and mental state of the mother. Other pathologists truly believed that respiratory infection was the underlying cause of death and today many pathologists still hold this view, with some justification. Though it is now generally thought that the infection is the trigger rather than the underlying cause, there is no doubt that some mild inflammatory condition of the air passages is implicated in a large proportion of SIDS.

Whether the pathologist really believed it or not, the practice grew up in the 1940s and 1950s of using terms such as acute bronchiolitis, acute tracheobronchitis or acute capillary bronchitis in the cot deaths where no specific pathological abnormalities could be found. In a proportion of these, subsequent microscopic examination reinforced the opinion of the pathologist that this was at least a contribution to the death, if not the whole cause.

There were, however, some disadvantages to this method of certification. First, the great variation in nomenclature meant that it was impossible to obtain statistics for research purposes. As there are true conditions (usually in sick children who do not die suddenly and unexpectedly) which go by these names, there was a mixture in the statistics of the SIDS and real respiratory infection. This meant that both classes were confused in the official figures, to the confusion of research workers and statisticians trying to assess various components of infant mortality.

There was another disadvantage in the use of these respiratory disease names for SIDS: the parents learned of the cause of death on the certificate and not unnaturally assumed that acute bronchiolitis was the same as 'acute bronchitis'. As it is well known that true chest infections such as severe bronchitis or pneumonia, especially in adults, are eminently treatable with antibiotics, the parents of some SIDS not unnaturally said 'Uncle Fred had pneumonia last year. The doctor gave him penicillin and he was as right as rain inside a week. Why didn't the doctor give my baby antibiotics for its acute bronchiolitis?' Of course, the child probably did not have acute bronchiolitis – certainly not in the true sense that many adults or older children get a severe chest infection due to bacteria rather than viruses. This misapprehension led a considerable number of parents to think that their doctor was incompetent or even negligent and one or two cases have occurred where the parents have taken legal action for medical negligence against the poor general practitioner. It is a fact that in some series of SIDS up to one third of the bereaved families have later changed their family doctor, apparently having lost faith in his abilities. This is naturally quite unjustified, as it is in other circumstances where the doctor is blamed for not anticipating death. For instance, a general practitioner may see a baby either in the surgery or at home during the winter, the parents complaining that the child has snuffles or diarrhoea. That child may die a cot death the next day and the parents will then blame the doctor for not recognising the child was so ill that it would die soon afterwards, but in a busy urban practice in the wintertime, the doctor may see half-a-dozen infants every day with signs of a cold or loose motions. The vast majority of these will *not* have a cot death – in fact, the average general practitioner only sees three or four SIDS in the whole of his career. It is therefore illogical, even if understandable, for the parents to blame the doctor for not foreseeing a fatality, when the victim of the later SIDS shows no different symptoms from scores of other children with trivial symptoms.

Let us return to the sequence of events after the tragedy has occurred: the cause of death given by the pathologist will be relayed to the coroner via his officer and, depending upon what actual wording the pathologist prefers to use, the consequences will differ. As already discussed, many pathologists in recent years use a term implying a respiratory infection, whether or not there is adequate evidence for it at the post-mortem examination. Unfortunately, there is still a residue of pathologists who are convinced that asphyxia and suffocation play a part in this syndrome. The numbers of these are declining rapidly, mainly due to retirement, but if a cause of death such as overlaying or suffocation by bedclothes or any cause suggesting some form of asphyxia is used, then the coroner has little option but to hold an inquest. In former years, inquests were held on virtually every case of SIDS, to the great distress of parents. Inquests on cot deaths are now very uncommon, not only because pathologists are more aware of the true nature of the syndrome, but because changes in the laws and rules governing coroners' procedures make inquests much less common in a whole range of deaths, but if a cause is given outright as some unnatural happening like overlaying or asphyxia, the coroner would have to have a theoretically public hearing to take verbal evidence from witnesses – in this case the parent or parents, though usually the medical evidence is now offered in documentary form.

Until a few years ago, these inquests were a full public performance, with local press reporters present. The tragedy would have been reported in the local newspapers, almost inevitably as 'mysterious death of baby' or some such description which increased the bewilderment of the parents and possibly aroused the suspicion of neighbours.

Some coroners a few years ago seem actually proud of the numbers of cot death inquests which they held, one at least appearing to think that he was performing some research function by giving such widespread publicity via his coroner's court.

Nowadays, the use of a cause of death referring to a chest infection, real or imagined, allows the coroner to write off the death as natural causes, issuing a death certificate on his pink 'Form B' which can be given to the registrar of births and deaths in the same way as an ordinary medical death certificate. The coroner often does this in the full knowledge of the pathologist's opinion on the true nature of cot death, and the legal fiction of spurious chest infections was commonly condoned by many coroners, especially those with medical qualifications.

Because of the disadvantages mentioned earlier the use of a term indicating a chest infection was discouraged in the late 1960s and in the early 1970s; the term sudden infant death syndrome was introduced by some doctors interested in the topic and was accepted after some campaigning by the Registrar-General, the Coroners' Society and the Royal College of Pathologists. Later on, in 1979, it was accepted internationally when the World Health Organisation gave it a separate category number (798.0) in the International Classification of Diseases, two large volumes devoted to the nomenclature of disease and causes of death.

Some pathologists, especially paediatric pathologists, however, quite legitimately object to the use of 'sudden infant death syndrome' on its own, saying that it is no better than using the words 'unknown' or 'unascertainable'. They feel that the description only reverts to the mysterious situation obtaining before respiratory infections were used as the cause of death, thus leaving the parents relatively unsatisfied. Many doctors do not agree with this criticism – including the author – as the term SIDS is now so well recognised by the international medical fraternity that it can hardly be mistaken for any other condition. True, it does not explain the underlying cause, but neither do the descriptions of many other diseases. Multiple sclerosis is a well-recognised and common disease, though the underlying cause is just as occult as that of cot death.

Some pathologists would rather sit on the fence – or hedge their bets – when giving a cause of death, in that they write something like 'acute bronchiolitis (sudden infant death syndrome)' indicating that they think it may be a respiratory infection but that the typical features make it a classical SIDS. As long as the cases are recognisable in the statistics and do not cause any social and personal hardship, the rather controversial matter of naming the cause of death is somewhat academic. The prime object is to remove any wording which could be construed as unnatural, as this leads to an investigation, sometimes in public, which only reinforces the grief and self-recrimination of the parents.

3 · What causes it?

One of the major factors which makes the sudden infant death syndrome so tragic is the aura of uncertainty which surrounds the cause, a feature which is particularly hard for bereaved parents to bear. Of the many comments made by both mothers and fathers the most frequent is that the lack of any definite reason for the death offered by their doctors was one of the hardest things to bear.

In literally hundreds of newspaper and magazine articles cot death has been given the name 'mystery' which in some ways has tended to perpetuate the sinister and occult nature of the condition. It is true that we still do not know why about 1 in 500 babies die in their sleep, but the mode or mechanism of death is becoming clearer and recent work holds out some hope of understanding the condition, which is the first step towards prevention.

The condition of SIDS must be distinguished from a true disease. It is called the sudden infant death *syndrome* which means that it is a recognisable set of circumstances, though without any evidence of a single, constant cause, such as is found in smallpox or tuberculosis.

As with most diseases of uncertain origin, theories abound and, at the time of writing, well over 2000 references in medical journals exist on the subject.

For many years, people were content to believe that sudden infant death was an unnatural condition caused by obstruction of the air passages leading to asphyxia. As already discussed, this was the origin of the overlaying theory, followed by misapprehensions about infant faces being buried in soft pillows, heavy bedclothes and the like. Stomach contents in the air passages were also a common certified cause of death, though there is no evidence that this is the cause, rather than an agonal change during the dying process. About one-quarter of all post-mortem examinations, both adult and child, reveal stomach contents in greater or lesser degree in the air passages, obvious evidence that it cannot be the *cause* in every case, but an *effect*.

If it is accepted that the sudden infant death syndrome is a process without any accidental mechanical mechanism, but a natural phenomenon within the body itself, then there is a very wide range of theories to be considered.

The mode of death is not a mystery in that it seems quite clear that the infants die of cardiorespiratory failure during sleep. This means that the heart stops, almost certainly as a result of failure of the breathing mechanism to deliver oxygen and remove waste carbon dioxide. Therefore the basic mechanism of death is respiratory failure. There is some argument as to whether this is central, that is failure of the controlling brain centres to maintain breathing, or obstructive, the closure of the air passages at the level of the throat or back of the mouth.

Whatever the mechanism, it now seems obvious that there is no single cause of cot death. There is no particular virus which kills small babies, there is no metabolic disease which is the root cause and no solitary agent can be incriminated, as in infectious diseases from viruses or bacteria.

It is now considered by almost everyone interested in the subject that SIDS is a *multi-factorial* disorder – in other words there are several factors which come together in a given baby at a given time and cause death (Fig. 10).

We know some of the factors but not others. Sleep and the age group seem virtually constant factors which have to be present. Up to half the cases have some type of infection, usually of the respiratory tract. There must be other factors, linked to the fact that cot death is more common in babies which were premature and underweight at birth. Many of the risk factors, which will be discussed later, found on statistical analysis of large numbers of SIDS, cannot be directly tied in to the individual case in terms of factors of the

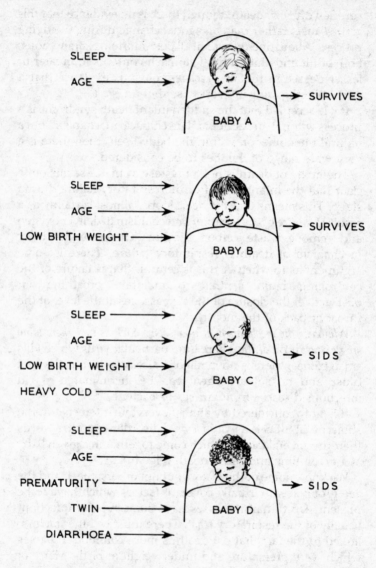

Fig. 10 The multi-factorial theory: on a given night, different babies may have different factors operating upon them. A minority may die, though not necessarily from the same factors

multi-factorial cause. For instance, it is hard to see how the marked social incidence or the mother's blood group can be incorporated in any model of causation, but this at present is merely an index of our ignorance of the subject.

If a multi-factorial cause is assumed it would seem that many babies suffer a number of these factors at any given time, but do not die. In a city on a night in winter there might be a dozen babies with three factors acting on them, half-a-dozen with four, three with five factors, but only one child with six operating on it – and that child might die a cot death.

Probably some of the 'near-misses', which will be discussed later, are babies who have either the full complement of adverse factors or almost that number, but one must not assume either that the number of factors necessary for SIDS is the same in every case or that the nature of the factors is constant. SIDS is a *final common pathway*, almost certainly via respiratory failure leading to heart failure and this pathway can be reached by a number of different routes. In the present poor state of knowledge, all we can do is to assess as many factors as we can discover and reject theories which cannot possibly fit the known pattern of SIDS victims.

The constitution of the child

Before coming to specific theories concerning either external influences like infections or dietary deficiencies or particular internal defects like glands or breathing control, we must consider some interesting, if shadowy, facts about the general constitution of babies who seem most at risk to SIDS. These characteristics have been discovered either by detailed retrospective enquiries about victims or by the examination of the 'near-misses', babies who were apparently in the throes of dying a cot death, but who were seen and revived in time.

Premature and low birth-weight infants are at increased risk of cot death, though the danger is still small in numerical terms. Whereas there are 7 per cent of such babies among all

new-born, 15 per cent of SIDS are small and/or premature. By
the time the danger period is reached at three to six months,
most will have caught up. Indeed, some pathologists have
said that their mental picture of the typical victim is that of a
somewhat plump male infant. Be that as it may, most of the
numerous surveys have shown that babies born before the
full nine-month term of pregnancy and those which are
significantly below the normal birth-weight appear more
often than expected in the records of SIDS. This may well be a
major part of the increased risk for twins, which are
characteristically small, early births.

Prematurity and low birth-weight, which naturally often
go hand-in-hand, mean that a more immature child is
launched on a separate existence. Many organs and tissues
are less ready for existing outside the comfortable environment of the mother's womb. The brain, for instance, does not
have the insulating myelin sheath around many of its nerve
fibres for many months after birth and a premature infant has
that much longer again with an immature nervous system,
which controls breathing and many other functions such as
heat regulation.

Some recent observations on SIDS and fragile babies are
interesting in this respect. It was found that the rate of cot
deaths was much higher among babies who had been in
special intensive care units after birth. The infant mortality in
all causes of death was much higher in these babies, being no
less than 44 per 1000 births, 10 times the rate in the general
population. Of these, 10 per cent were SIDS, making the rate
for cot deaths 4.4 per 1000 births, much higher – about
twice – the usual rate. This high mortality rate was for babies
up to 11 months, long after they had been discharged from
the neonatal special care units, showing that the delicate hold
on life, usually associated with prematurity and immaturity,
led to some long-lasting fragility and susceptibility to SIDS.
The authors of this study (Kulkarni and others) commented
that among these infants, who seemed well at the time of
their discharge from hospital and at subsequent examination,
SIDS and deaths from infections constituted the largest

proportion of deaths in the post-neonatal period, i.e., after one week of age. They concluded that the factors that appeared to be important in the birth of high-risk infants continued to be operative in the post-neonatal period and contributed to the high mortality. Many other articles in medical literature in recent years emphasise this relationship between intra-uterine and perinatal factors in the causation of sudden infant deaths later in infancy.

Another related fact was reported from Seattle, a place very active in SIDS research. This was that SIDS was more common where a short interval existed between pregnancies – a young mother who had a succession of babies relatively quickly was more likely to have a SIDS among them. The authors of the paper found that this also increased the risk of deaths immediately after birth and of congenital defects; they ascribed the cause to low birth-weight where babies come close together.

Studies mainly in the United States have built evidence to show that babies who suffer crib deaths or 'near-misses' are different in many ways to control babies, though many paediatricians would dispute this. These workers challenge the common view that most SIDS babies are quite well before the tragedy, though the differences often seem to be of behaviour, rather than of illness. For example, there is considerable interest in the *cry* of a high-risk baby, which has been analysed for the sound content, as well as being described generally. It is said that the sounds were weaker, of shorter duration and breathy, being of higher pitch, with abrupt changes in pitch. One of the world's most active researchers into SIDS, Dr Steinschneider of the University of Maryland, is carrying out a large-term investigation which includes much probing into respiratory functions. He has confirmed that there are often differences in the cry of the potential and 'near-miss' crib death infant and has even found lesser changes of a similar nature in the siblings (brothers and sisters) of infants at risk.

Other characteristics of the potential victim have been described, but they are treated with extreme caution by most researchers and paediatricians. It has been suggested that SIDS babies were less active and reactive to their environment than controls; they reacted less to stimuli and became more breathless and exhausted during feeding. The criticisms of this sort of observation revolve around the non-specificity and the possibility of misuse of the data if publicised irresponsibly; it is pointed out that 37 per cent of all babies can be classified as less active and 6 per cent are extremely passive and unreactive, yet SIDS attacks only 0.2 per cent of the infant population. As a predictive method this approach is obviously useless and possibly harmful if misunderstood by parents and the general media.

Is there a 'cause' of SIDS?

To return to the main-stream of research and theories about cot death: it seems essential to clarify our ideas about what we mean by the cause. As mentioned earlier, most workers now agree that there is no single, as yet undiscovered, reason for SIDS. For many years research has been bedevilled and perhaps retarded by a mistaken notion that some obscure virus lurks in the victims or some specific biochemical defect exists in the body processes. Very few now believe this and most would agree that it is a multi-factorial syndrome. The final tragedy of a sudden infant death is the final common pathway – almost certainly an eventual failure of respiration and heart beat – which is the terminal mechanism by which life becomes extinct. The intermediate and initiating processes remain obscure and are now the target for intensive research, especially by the physiologists concerned with breathing control and circulatory responses.

We must not assume that the number of factors is always the same to arrive at a fatal outcome – the nature of the factors, as well as their total number, may be different in different cases. It must again be emphasised that SIDS is the outward manifestation of deranged internal bodily functions, but these need not be the same derangements in each fatality. It is the final common event that we see but, in the present state of knowledge, we have little or no means of knowing how individual babies reached the tragic end. More and more, child health doctors and pathologists are accepting that the whole concept of SIDS is a much more variable and fluid event in terms of underlying causes than was previously thought – that is why it is futile and perhaps cruel to expect a sudden breakthrough, so beloved of journalists, which will prevent SIDS, literally overnight, in the way that antibiotics cured pneumonias or global vaccination has eradicated smallpox. In the present state of knowledge, all we can do is to investigate as many factors as we can find and reject theories which cannot possibly fit the known pattern of SIDS.

What are the past and present theories about SIDS?

When the causes of a disease are not known, theories abound. A prime example was diabetes, which had a mythology all of its own until the role of the pancreas and insulin was discovered. Similarly, the obscure nature of sudden infant death, which is so reluctant to yield its secrets, has given rise to a proliferation of hypotheses and theories. Many can be discarded with little hesitation, as they just cannot be moulded to fit the pattern of SIDS; others, at first sight unlikely candidates in themselves, may fit into the jigsaw of the multifactorial situation we have discussed. It seems clear now that different cases of cot death have arrived at the fatal common pathway via different initial routes and some of the theories may fit some cases but not others.

The number of speculative ideas is vast – a search of the medical literature at the time of writing this book yielded over 2000 articles either wholly or partly about SIDS. Every month, a new idea is sprung upon the medical world, apart from all the more routine articles which are doggedly pursuing the more conventional pathways of research. Unfortunately, the popular press constantly seizes on these and a press-cutting service is kept hard at work extracting hundreds of articles all reporting – or even blazoning – a new breakthrough, which usually is never heard of again. These over-emphatic and often ill-understood reports do nothing to help and often cause heartache and distress to cot-death parents, who read into them some element of self-reproach, partly through misreporting and partly misunderstanding. The Foundation for the Study of Infant Deaths in London often has to take issue with bad reporting of this type, which either upsets parents or gives rise to unjustified hopes of instant prevention.

It must be said, of course, that there is a great deal in the medical journals that is sound, sometimes brilliant research, which may clarify our knowledge of infant physiology and pathology – and even if it leads to no advance in the understanding of the causes of SIDS, it may equally well cut off yet another blind alley, saving the efforts of future workers in the same futile direction.

Some of the very many ideas which were or still are current include the following:

ALLERGY TO COW'S MILK

One of the early classical research projects in the really scientific phase of SIDS investigation was that into the possibility that cot deaths were an allergic response to foreign protein in the form of cow's milk. In the late 1950s and early 1960s, work in Cambridge and London suggested that a model of SIDS could be produced in guinea-pigs. Allergic responses occur when, after one dose of a foreign protein, the body defences begin to produce antibodies which neutralise any subsequent entry of the same protein, but often with dramatic symptoms during the neutralisation reaction. When cow's milk was introduced into the windpipes of normal, unsensitised guinea-pigs, nothing happened, but if the animals had been sensitised to cow's milk by previous injections spaced out over a few weeks, the entry of milk into their windpipes caused a violent reaction and often death, quite unlike SIDS. If the guinea-pigs were lightly anaesthetised by drugs to simulate sleep, the introduction of a few drops of milk over the tongue into the larynx and windpipe caused a quiet death very similar to SIDS. In addition, it was thought at that time that some microscopical changes in the lungs and small air passages, with loosening of the lining of the bronchi, were similar to that seen in post-mortem samples from SIDS victims, though this appearance is now considered to be an artefact.

The findings caused considerable interest and even excitement at the time. Even today, many researchers wonder if there might be some element of truth as at least a partial explanation of SIDS. Although further work showed that SIDS victims did have cow's-milk antibodies in their blood, it was also shown that non-SIDS babies also had them. The theory could not explain the age and seasonal nor social class differences, nor the variation in twins. One big flaw was that babies develop cow's-milk antibodies very quickly and early in life, during the first weeks or even days, yet SIDS is characteristically most dangerous at two to five months. So why should this mechanism, which depends on cow's-milk feeding, be worse at a time when the child is beginning to move on to other types of food?

Another problem was that at the time it was thought that all SIDS occurred in bottle-fed (i.e. cow's milk) babies and never in breast-fed babies. This has now been shown to be untrue and numerous cases of totally breast-fed SIDS victims are on record. The saga of cow's-milk allergy is still not closed, but is no longer held to be a likely explanation in the search for an answer, in the majority of cases.

VIRUS INFECTIONS

Another strong contender in the field of theories is the infection by viruses as a cause of SIDS. Here we have a double issue. First, the possibility of an overwhelming virus infection as the one and only cause of death: or a role for a respiratory infection by viruses as a 'trigger' or partial cause of the syndrome . . . in other words, one of the factors of our multi-factorial situation.

The fortunes of the total theory tend to wax and wane. There are enthusiastic protagonists of the idea, usually expert virologists or microbiologists who claim to be able to grow specific viruses in a significant proportion of SIDS cases. One such virus is the respiratory syncytial virus (RS virus), which has been accused of causing the whole SIDS problem. It is true that RS virus is a common cause of respiratory disease in children, some of whom die, though rarely in the sudden unexpected way of SIDS. The problem is that few pathologists and virologists have been able to detect RS or any other virus in SIDS autopsy material with any degree of constancy.

As so often happens in medical research, only the enthusiasts are able to substantiate their own claims to any great degree. This is not a criticism, but is due to a number of factors, not least the fact that they may be far more expert in a particular technique than anyone else. But, as in all cot death research, workers are bedevilled by the disadvantage of having to carry out all tests retrospectively – and trying to isolate viruses and culture micro-organisms from post-mortem material is a difficult and uncertain task. Many workers have isolated a wide variety of viruses and bacteria from SIDS cases, but no one is yet convinced that the random and inconstant results really add up to any real conclusion. This is partly due to the loss of virus after death, after refrigeration of the tissues and the common problem of contamination of post-mortem material. No proof of a well-established virus infection in the tissues is forthcoming, such as accumulation of inflammatory cells in the lungs or air passages, though the protagonists of the virus theory say that this is because the speed of the infection is so rapid and overwhelming that death occurs before any signs have time to appear. So far, this claim has failed to make much impression on the rather sceptical main body of opinion in the research world.

It is true that up to half the cases of SIDS have a history of some illness in preceding days, often a hint or actual sign of a respiratory infection. Coupled with the possibility of blocked nasal passages and perhaps a brainstem affectation by circulating viruses, the theory would fit in well with a partial contribution of such an infection to the multi-factorial explanation, to which we shall return later. There is so far quite insufficient evidence to say that any specific virus or bacteria kills in SIDS by a direct infective disease.

CALCIUM METABOLISM

One possible explanation for the respiratory failure mode of death in SIDS (especially the so-called 'obstructive' apnoea element to be described later) is the mechanical closure of the upper air passages by spasm of the larynx at the level of the vocal cords. It has also been pointed out that the very common and profuse pin-point haemorrhages on the surface of the lungs may be due to efforts to breathe against a closed larynx.

This condition of spasm of the vocal cords is sometimes seen quite apart from SIDS in a condition called 'tetany', due to a lack of calcium in the blood. Low calcium makes the muscles everywhere in the body very irritable and cramps and spasms may occur. (This must not be confused with 'tetanus', a very serious infective disease, but the common name is due to severe muscle spasms that occur in both conditions.) In tetany, which can occur in several conditions where calcium metabolism is abnormal, such as rickets or certain kidney diseases, the muscles of the voice box (larynx) can go into spasm and the two vocal cords can come across the airway, blocking it completely. The calcium levels in the blood are controlled to a large extent by four tiny glands in the neck, called the parathyroids and it was postulated some years ago in Scandinavia that SIDS infants had an abnormal development of their parathyroids. A Danish researcher found that there were fewer such glands in the necks of SIDS infants and alleged that they also had abnormalities in the calcium level of their serum measured after post-mortem.

Repetition of his work by several other researchers in Britain and America, however, showed that the missing glands were usually lurking in the upper part of the chest, having not reached their adult position in the neck. The changes in the calcium levels – always of doubtful significance like most post-mortem chemical analyses – could not be verified and the theory fell into oblivion, but other workers still have thoughts about calcium metabolism in more general terms. The joint between the ends of the ribs and the cartilage joining them to the breast bone (sternum) sometimes give microscopical evidence of some defect in calcium metabolism in SIDS, though this may be an index of a period of ill-health which was clinically unsuspected. Laryngeal spasm, unassociated with calcium defects, has been revived as a possible contribution to breathing problems, as will be described later.

MAGNESIUM DEFICIENCY

A more recent theory from the United States alleges that magnesium levels in the blood of SIDS are low and that this can cause or contribute to death by its well-known effect on the stability of contraction of the heart muscle. Though, as in many theories, the evidence is quite impressive, there are the usual problems of fitting such a hypothesis into the known epidemiological pattern of SIDS and so far the idea has failed to gain widespread acceptance.

VITAMIN E DEFICIENCY

A quite unsuccessful theory was that vitamin E or pantothenic acid, found in wheat germ and other vegetable sources, was related to SIDS. The necessity for this vitamin has never been satisfactorily proved in humans and the idea has not gained any credence.

SELENIUM DEFICIENCY

Like the last theory, the deficiency in this rare element was a poor starter in the SIDS hypothesis range.

SPINAL HAEMORRHAGES

A pathologist in the United States claimed that a considerable proportion of crib deaths that he had investigated had had haemorrhages into the spinal canal, a place normally not examined in any detail, but his work has not been confirmed by several other pathologists who began looking there and the reason for this alleged finding remains a mystery; it may have been a post-mortem artefact, due to settling of blood into the spinal canal after death.

LOW TEMPERATURE – HYPOTHERMIA

A low environmental temperature and a subsequent drop in body temperature (hypothermia) has been put forward as a possibility on several occasions. Some of the earlier work came from Canada, where naturally very low winter temperatures are seen. However, most SIDS occur where the possibility of hypothermia is highly unlikely or even impossible. It occurs in Mediterranean and tropical countries where the climates make it virtually impossible for cold to be a factor, though admittedly statistics on SIDS are usually very poor in these areas. It is true that seasonally most SIDS occur in the winter months, but most experts would consider that extreme periods of cold weather do not seem to be associated with an increase in SIDS. When this is carefully tested, it may not be so clear-cut and there seems to be some statistical correlation between changes in the weather and the rate of SIDS, even though those changes are not gross in terms of temperature drop.

The present writer was co-author of a paper which related meteorological conditions in South Wales to the incidence of cot deaths over a considerable number of years. There was a definite statistical relationship between the rate and the temperature, though naturally no individual connection in any particular SIDS case could be detected. Incidentally, the same investigation showed that there were more SIDS when there was an epidemic of influenza A type in the community, but not when influenza B was prevalent. Even so, the relation of influenza was slight, accounting for only about 5 per cent of the difference in SIDS incidence.

To return to the effect of weather: the past impressions of many pathologists were that SIDS seemed more prevalent in or after cool, damp weather rather than cold 'snaps' and certainly the impression remains that hard, icy conditions do not seem at all related to an increase in cot deaths.

To show the inconsistency and contradictions in medical theorising, it has even been argued that the very opposite may be related to SIDS, where a child is kept in too warm a place and perhaps with too many cot coverings.

CARBON DIOXIDE POOLING

One theory was current for a time, that the gas carbon dioxide (not to be confused with carbon monoxide from gas heaters, fires and exhausts) might accumulate around the infant and cause suffocation. Carbon dioxide is a very heavy gas and collects at lower levels. It is exhaled in the breath and the hypothesis was that it might sink back around the baby and gradually accumulate in conditions where it could not escape. If the sides of the sleeping place were impervious, such as a carry-cot with plastic sides, the level of the heavy gas would gradually climb until it surrounded the baby's head and caused oxygen lack by depriving it of the lighter gas, oxygen.

This theory was again found untenable as most SIDS occur in physical situations where this is impossible and no entrapment of carbon dioxide could occur. For instance, in the common type of cot with bars or slats at the side, the heavy gas would simply run out and disperse around the floor. Even in a carry-cot, it is highly unlikely that the dioxide would settle into a static layer as draughts in the room and convection currents from the warmth of the baby would so mix up the gases that the pooling of an appreciable amount would be remote. Apart from that, the theory totally fails to fit in with the pattern of age, season, social class, twinning, etc., and can be discounted as a candidate for serious consideration.

HEART CONDUCTION DEFECTS

This is entering a very specialised and medically technical area where controversy has gone this way and that for a number of years. There is no doubt that near-miss infants, who narrowly escape dying from SIDS, tend to have a high incidence of cardiac abnormalities in terms of physiological testing. Slow heart rates and abnormal electrical traces on electrocardiograms (ECG) have been described in great detail. In addition, pathologists working on minute details of the heart structure from tissues recovered at post-mortem examination have found frequent abnormalities, though their significance is disputed. The heart beat is paced by two small nodules of specialised muscle fibres, from which conducting fibres spread out through the heart muscle to control the rhythm. These nodules and fibres are in turn modulated by the autonomic nervous system coming from the brain and spinal cord. Several researchers have claimed that the nodules and the bundles of conducting fibres are distorted or partly replaced by inert fibrous tissue in many SIDS victims. It is not possible to correlate the undoubted functional abnormalities in the near-miss babies with the observed structural defects and, indeed, the latter are said by other experts to be merely remodelling changes which occur in babies normally and which are not pathological.

Similar changes occur in the kidneys; a former claim that up to 15 per cent of the kidney glomeruli were fibrosed in SIDS was shown to be a normal change in all babies.

The functional abnormalities which are now beyond doubt are also hard to evaluate in terms of cause or effect. Heart changes can occur from oxygen deficiency which, as shown below, is thought to be caused by breathing troubles. So, are the heart changes primary and a cause of SIDS, or are they secondary to diffuse damage caused by oxygen lack from respiratory defects? This area is the most active under investigation at present, and it is hoped that a few years will provide the answer.

HOUSE MITE ALLERGY

A fairly recent, but not generally credited, theory is based on the assumption that SIDS may be due to allergy to the foreign protein of house mites. These tiny creatures, widely found in house dust in the cleanest of homes, are undoubtedly responsible for some forms of allergic complaints, including skin rashes and a form of asthma. There seems no possibility, though, that they form any substantial element in SIDS but, in view of our contention that many different factors might contribute in different fatal episodes, we cannot summarily dismiss any theory as being occasionally a trigger or precipitating factor.

BACTERIAL INFECTION

Even less than the virus infection hypothesis, bacterial diseases seem non-starters in the present state of knowledge about sudden infant death. For many years, although the investigations at a post-mortem examination on a SIDS victim have included the taking of a sample for bacterial culture – or 'microbiological investigation' in modern terminology – no constantly recurring organism or germ has been found. Once again, the problems of retrospective investigation after death make the interpretation of any findings very difficult. Many bacteria and other micro-organisms die soon after the death of the body and some are destroyed by refrigeration, which usually precedes the autopsy and may be delayed a day or so. Where many bacteria grow on laboratory culture from samples, it can be difficult to know which were contaminants at or after death and which were merely sitting in the tissues but not causing any disease, as inert carrier-states are common. No specific organism has been accused of SIDS; the small proportion of babies who die rapidly contain a few who have a genuine pneumonia and these may yield the causative organism, be it virus or bacteria, on culture in the laboratory. However, these then by definition cease to be included in the true SIDS group.

BOTULISM

As a sequel to the last item about bacterial infections, one possible cause has been advanced several times over the years and some recent articles in the medical press have revived some interest in the subject. This is the notion that botulism may be involved. Botulism is an illness, often fatal, caused by a toxin produced by the botulinus organism, a form of food poisoning. The botulinus toxin is one of the most poisonous substances known to man, a minute fraction of a milligram being sufficient to cause death. It grows in the intestine and the toxin can be absorbed into the bloodstream. In recent years, some routine investigations after a SIDS autopsy have revealed the presence of the botulinus organism in the intestine. These cases were mostly in California, though other sporadic reports have come from elsewhere.

It is very difficult to evaluate the significance of this finding. Undoubtedly the vast majority of SIDS deaths have no relation at all to botulism and it is hard to see how it could fit the set pattern of age, social class, season, etc. However, once again we cannot close our minds to any theory or contribution and it might as well be that a small proportion of SIDS may have this particular infection as yet another of the multiple factors that add up to a fatal result. Some 4 per cent of crib deaths investigated in California in a year revealed the presence of botulism. The infants showed weakness, feeding troubles, constipation and a lack of sucking and crying ability due to muscular weakness. There may be a link here, as they seemed to have the same weakness affecting their breathing and airway muscles, which may in turn be related to the respiratory failure described below as the current best theory of causation. Botulism may come from many sources such as house dust, soil or sometimes honey. American doctors impressed by the evidence about botulism have actually recommended the avoidance of honey for babies under one year of age; after this age even honey with botulism organisms appears to be safe because the intestines of older children and adults can deal with it.

STRESS

A very non-specific title, this concept of stress was one of the older theories of SIDS. It was current 20 or so years ago when cortisone and the hormones of the adrenal glands were very much in the news. Stress of any sort in adults – from traffic injuries to surgical operations – can reduce the amount of lipoid in the adrenal cortex and the amount of circulating hormones, but in infants there is little evidence that this is anything to do with SIDS. Infections are a form of stress and these can deplete the supply of steroids from the adrenal glands. Some researchers have described abnormalities in SIDS adrenals, probably related to infection, but again it is hard to disentangle cause and effect. Several organs, including the spleen and the thymus gland, show alterations in many infant diseases, especially where the illness has been prolonged or where there is a diffuse infection. In fact, some SIDS have been shown to have been ill for longer than their lack of obvious symptoms would suggest, by the finding of these stress changes in the organs on very careful examination with the microscope.

But are these related to the cause of the death or are they merely an index of a baby that has not been very well? Of course, in the multi-factorial situation, the two are inter-related and we find ourselves forced to agree that sudden infant death is not a specific, single disease, but the end result of a very variable pathway.

INFANTICIDE

This can be disposed of very quickly and definitely. One rather uncritical medical writer claimed that all crib deaths were really hidden homicides! The claim is so fatuous as to be disregarded out of hand, but it can do harm to the campaign to reassure families and mothers that there is no element of self-blame or recrimination in the cause of SIDS. Of course, one cannot go to the other extreme and dismiss every infant death as natural causes without any investigation. This is why all sudden infant deaths must be reported to the coroner, medical examiner or similar authority, to exclude the very few criminal or grossly negligent deaths that admittedly do occur. Unfortunately, the need for this screening process itself causes confusion among some people, who associate the involvement of the coroner with child abuse or infanticide.

The post-mortem examination is all important in this matter and though a natural reluctance and even revulsion at the idea is understandable, it is vital for two reasons: (a) to exclude any criminal or unnatural cause, for everyone's reassurance and peace of mind and (b) to try to arrive at the true cause of death, both for that particular victim and to further the vital course of research.

ERRORS OF METABOLISM

There are several well-known diseases of children due to an inborn error of metabolism, defects in the chemistry of the body, usually in the processing of various food substances. Most of these illnesses are recognised early in childhood and under treatment, so the picture is most unlike SIDS, where a virtually well infant suddenly dies. There is no evidence that such a defect occurs in cot deaths. Most of the illnesses are familial or hereditary, passed on by one or other of the parents, and may run in whole families. Thankfully, this does not happen in SIDS and there is no evidence at all of a family trait in sudden infant death. As mentioned earlier, where press reports of multiple cot deaths are seen, it is very likely that some familial metabolic disease is present, even if it is not recognised at the time.

FAILURE OF THE IMMUNITY SYSTEM

Some infants have a congenital absence of the special immune proteins in their blood which protect against infection. These unfortunates may have to spend much time in sterile surroundings and be carefully protected against infections. It was tempting to think of some parallel with SIDS and earlier theories worked along these lines. It was known that many SIDS had a mild infection and that there was much discussion about the death being due to an overwhelming virus or bacterial infection, before the body could marshal its defences.

A major part of such defences lies in the immunity system. The proteins in the blood carrying the antibodies that fight infections are the gamma-globulins and it was postulated that perhaps SIDS victims had none or too little of these globulins. The theory was attractive in that it might explain why cot death struck mostly around two to six months and not nearer birth, because this was when the immunity passed on by the mother was on the wane, yet the baby had not yet developed its own active immunity from challenges by micro-organisms. Unfortunately, no real proof of hypogammaglo-bulinaemia, the term describing low protective proteins, is forthcoming in the post-mortem material on SIDS babies.

LUNG SURFACTANT

A very recent line of research being conducted in Britain concerns a substance in the lungs called 'surfactant'. Because of the tiny size of the terminal air spaces in the lungs, the moist surfaces and the huge total area, the physical properties of the walls of these air spaces make them adhere together very strongly. A good analogy is that of a damp plastic bag, where it can be very difficult to pull apart the two sides when the bag is folded flat. In the normal lung, a chemical is produced by the lining cells which markedly lowers the surface tension, so allowing the walls to separate. If it were not for this substance, surfactant, the slight negative pressure available for breath-ing, produced when the chest wall expands and the diaphragm descends, would not be sufficient to allow air to expand the lungs.

Dr Colin Morley, of Cambridge, while measuring surfactant in different groups of babies (as it was known to be deficient in premature infants who suffered from a breathing disorder known as the 'respiratory distress syndrome') found almost accidentally that SIDS victims had both less surfactant and abnormal surfactant. He is currently receiving a grant from the Foundation for the Study of Infant Deaths to pursue this research and to try to devise a method for detecting surfactant deficiency in live babies, rather than in post-mortem samples. At present, it is not known whether the surfactant changes in SIDS occur a long time before death, shortly before the tragedy or even as a post-mortem change.

SODIUM AND ELECTROLYTES – HYPERNATRAEMIA

Earlier, we mentioned the theory that calcium and magnesium might be involved in SIDS, though the proof was unacceptably thin. Another electrolyte – a metallic molecule or ion in the body fluids – is vital to the proper stability of the internal environment. This is sodium, derived mostly from the intake of salt. It is closely bound up with the retention of water in the tissues, though this is a gross oversimplification. In the fluid part of the body – which is by far the greater part of it – there is an exquisitely balanced proportion of small molecules such as sodium, potassium, calcium, magnesium, etc. Any upset of the ratios, especially involving sodium and potassium, may cause profound disturbances, with either waterlogging (oedema), or dehydration or disturbances of heart contraction. When sodium is lost through the kidneys, water is also lost with it and the child becomes dehydrated. In severe cases, an intravenous infusion (drip) of saline or other special electrolytic fluids is needed.

The relevance of all this to sudden infant death is that some years ago, especially in the SIDS research centre at Sheffield, it was discovered that some infant victims, though they appeared superficially well during the few days before death, were overloaded with sodium; this was ascribed to excessive feeding with too concentrated National Dried Milk, the baby formula issued by the Health Service clinics. Some mothers, with the best intentions, had been 'overscooping' the powder when mixing the feed. That particular type of food was rich in sodium and when the children either fell slightly ill for other reasons such as an infection – or when they reacted adversely to the feed, the mothers thought that they were hungry and gave them yet more food and more sodium. What the children really needed was plain water, to dilute the feed and wash out the sodium in their urine. This sodium overload is called hypernatraemia.

At the time, there was a flurry of excitement at the possible identification of the cause of cot death, but it seemed to be a relatively isolated phenomenon and, once recognised, was soon overcome. In fact, the expert team at Sheffield, led by Professor John Emery, recently published another article drawing attention to the fact that this danger seemed to have faded by 1979 from the peak period of 1971–2. This was attributed to better education about infant feeding as well as some modification in the composition of the milk powder. A reduction in infantile diarrhoea – which itself causes hypernatraemia from loss of body water – and an increased incidence of breast feeding, were also suggested as reasons for the reduction of this condition. In 1974, it was reported that 172 out of 302 Sheffield mothers (57 per cent) prepared over-concentrated feeds, but health education there has made a marked impact on this particular danger.

Once again, though this problem of hypernatraemia may have been one of the elements in our multi-factorial situation, we certainly cannot look to it for anything more than a fragmentary part of the whole spectrum of sudden infant death.

THE CONTROL OF RESPIRATION – SLEEP APNOEA

Now we come to the theory – or rather, the inter-related group of theories – which at the present time hold the most promise of explaining the sudden infant death syndrome. These revolve around the complex physiological control of breathing, especially during sleep. Now that recent research has turned away from the simplistic idea of a single cause for SIDS, the most exciting current work is that which concerns sleep apnoea, the control of breathing and associated functions.

First, the actual mode of death has to be defined further. The mode of death means the way in which life terminates. This in itself partly depends upon definitions of death, but in SIDS the problems of definition are not so controversial as in the long-standing arguments about brain death in relation to organ transplantation.

Death, in the usual meaning of the word, takes place when the functions of the brain, heart and lungs cease. In adult natural deaths, there is usually a chain reaction by which each of these major systems fails one after the other. For example, if a man has a coronary heart attack, the heart may stop, which means that the brain is immediately deprived of blood. In a matter of moments the nervous control of breathing will cease, so respiration stops and brain death itself follows within a few minutes. If by immediate resuscitative measures such as cardiac massage the heart is started again, then brain function and breathing are restored.

Most deaths are primarily cardiac in origin because the heart fails. The lungs and brain fail as a secondary result of this heart failure. Sometimes, the brain may fail primarily, as in a large cerebral haemorrhage or in severe head injury. In these cases, the heart and lungs may function for a very long time, though if the brain damage is severe, respiration stops next and eventually the heart ceases because no oxygen is being provided by the failed respiratory system.

Primarily lung failure is less common, though it can occur because of waterlogging, infection or blockage by blood clot.

The relevance of all this to SIDS is that the immediate mode of death appears to be respiratory failure, that is, breathing ceases. Though there is one school of research which believes that there are primary abnormalities in the heart, most researchers feel that it is the brain-lung duet that is the way in which death occurs and that the heart stops because of the failure of respiration. All these functions are inextricably linked and it is very difficult to separate one from the other. In the currently favoured theory of the mechanism of SIDS, the sequence of events is thought to be as follows:

1. Certain infants have a tendency to prolonged sleep apnoea – known as PSA. Apnoea means absence of breathing and is a feature of everyone, both infant and adult. Especially during sleep, the regular rhythm of a child's breathing is broken so that cycles of normal speed breathing alternate with slow breathing, even to the point of complete cessation. It has been found in recent years that adults also have sleep apnoea, which may be prolonged in certain disease states such as high blood pressure. During sleep there are various levels of consciousness which are associated with rotatory eye movements, dreaming and other physiological changes. The breathing pattern also seems linked to these different depths of sleep.

All infants have some degree of sleep apnoea, but in most it is not prolonged sleep apnoea (PSA). If one listens to any small baby while asleep in its cot – and small infants can spend at least three-quarters of their lives asleep – the alternating rhythm of breathing can easily be noticed. The common use of baby alarms has made this evident: they provide an easy means for the parent to listen to the child's breathing. There tends to be a period of normal rhythmic breathing which then slows down until it ceases altogether. A few seconds follow in which no breaths are taken, then the breathing begins again and rapidly regains the normal pattern. This is repeated throughout the sleeping period, with variations according to the type of sleep being maintained (Fig. 11).

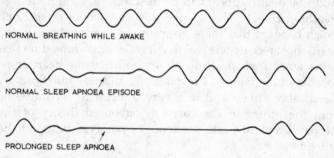

NORMAL BREATHING WHILE AWAKE

NORMAL SLEEP APNOEA EPISODE

PROLONGED SLEEP APNOEA

Fig. 11 Patterns of breathing

The control of breathing is from the respiratory nerve centres in the brainstem, which is the prolongation of the upper spinal cord just within the base of the skull. From here, nerves pass out through the base of the skull and travel down the neck into the chest. These are the vagus nerves, from the Greek for 'wanderer', as they pass down from the head through the chest and abdomen, carrying automatic (autonomic) nervous signals of which we are not normally aware.

During early infancy, it appears that this nervous control of breathing is unstable and does not establish a regular fixed pattern until near the end of the first year of life. That is the usual pattern of sleep in most infants, but a proportion of babies have PSA, that is longer periods of non-breathing between the normal regular cycles. The threshold for abnormality is rather uncertain, but a child who holds its breath in this way for more than 15 seconds is considered to have PSA.

2. During periods of PSA, there is naturally a deficiency of oxygen being taken into the bloodstream, one of the prime functions of the breathing apparatus being to absorb oxygen from the air and combine it with the haemoglobin of the blood for transport round the body. Thus there is a tendency for hypoxia (a deficiency of oxygen) to begin if sleep apnoea is unduly prolonged.

At the same time, carbon dioxide accumulates in the blood because the other function of breathing, apart from taking in oxygen, is to blow off the waste products of metabolism in the form of carbon dioxide.

The normal control of breathing is strongly linked with the levels of these two substances in the blood. The breathing centres in the brain are driven both by increase of carbon dioxide and decrease of oxygen. The relative importance of the two is a matter of great complexity and some argument, but is the reason why we cannot voluntarily hold our breath for very long as the lack of oxygen and the build-up of carbon dioxide over-ride our voluntary desire to refrain from breathing.

In some infants, it appears that this sensitivity to oxygen lack and carbon dioxide build-up is deficient. In some animals, such as seals, there is an in-built ability to ignore these signals because the animal needs to spend a long time under water. This is the so-called 'dive reflex' which enables a seal to spend up to 20 minutes without breathing, even though the chemical levels would have long forced other animals to restart respiration. It is considered that some infants have a parallel to this 'dive reflex', in that they do not respond either sufficiently or quickly enough to the chemical signals. The monitoring of this chemistry of the blood is done both in the respiratory centres in the brain and also in little collections of nerve endings in the carotid arteries in the neck.

3. It is considered that there is a circular effect between PSA and anoxia, so that once an anoxic state occurs because of PSA, that anoxia itself prolongs the apnoea and a descending spiral of respiratory activity begins. Several factors tend to encourage this to happen.

One such factor is the sleep itself, which depresses the activity of the respiratory centres. Virtually all SIDS victims die during sleep and it is also noticeable that most deaths occur early in the day, most of them in the early hours of the morning. This seems almost certainly related to the depth of sleep at this time, rather than perhaps the more shallow sleeping of daytime naps.

4. Virus infections act on this PSA-anoxia cycle in several ways. First, any viraemia (a virus infection throughout the body) tends to depress brain activity. No specific virus need be incriminated, but in the common cold and associated coryzal infections, there is undoubtedly a virus circulating in the blood and present in most organs. It need not be a very virulent virus and in itself is certainly not a fatal infection. The same may apply to some of the gastro-enteric viruses which are the cause of infantile diarrhoea.

In addition to this viraemia acting directly on the breathing centres in the brain, there is another effect of virus infection of the upper respiratory passages. In the ordinary snuffles or common cold, the mucous membrane lining of the nose, back of the throat and communication between the nasal cavities and the throat may become swollen and covered in mucus. The internal nasal and throat passages of an infant are very small indeed and even slight oedema (swelling) and mucus-covering will greatly reduce or even block the passage of air. We now have a situation where the shallow or absent respiratory movements are being aggravated by restriction of the passage of air, making the anoxia worse and therefore driving the circular mechanism around its descending spiral. Some infants are obligatory nose breathers at this age. This means that if their nose is partly blocked they have to make the best of it because they do not have the ability to breathe through their mouths. This has been shown in certain infants by gently closing the nostrils, pinching the nose with the fingers. The child then may become blue and in respiratory distress because no alternative route is provided by mouth breathing.

We now have a dynamic situation which is fraught with danger. The depressed brainstem centres become less ready to send nervous impulses to the chest muscles and diaphragm in order to restart breathing. The child is deeply asleep, is short of oxygen and is unresponsive to rise in

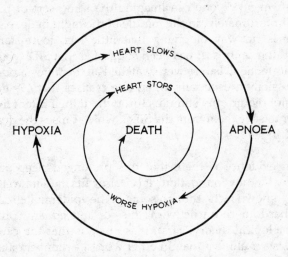

Fig. 12 Ondine's curse

carbon dioxide. A deepening state of hypoxia takes place and this can rapidly lead to sudden failure of the heart which is very dependent upon a constant good oxygen supply. It may well be that at this point, some of the alleged abnormalities in the conducting system of the heart muscle may play a secondary role.

The descending spiral or respiratory activity is sometimes called 'Ondine's Curse' and unless interrupted can lead to death (Fig. 12). In poliomyelitis – which significantly used to be called infantile paralysis – a similar situation arose because a specific virus, that of polio, attacked the brainstem specifically. The breathing centres were knocked out by the virus and until the invention of the iron lung, as it used to be called, death was virtually inevitable in severe bulbar polio. Marginal cases had a partial paralysis of respiratory centres and some of the old doctors still remember that patients 'forgot to breathe'. Sometimes their apnoea could be rapidly terminated by pinching the skin or otherwise stimulating them. The general stimulation of nerves gave the brain a little kick, which started the respiratory centres pulsing again. In SIDS, one can imagine the same sort of pattern but, unfortunately, in the middle of the night in deep sleep, there is no way of giving that little kick to re-start the breathing centres. It has been suggested that SIDS could be eradicated if all babies were watched all the time – a practical impossibility, especially when one realises that 499 infants will not require any stimulus throughout their infant lives in order to save them from the SIDS, which causes the death of the 1 in 500.

What evidence is there that this prolonged sleep apnoea theory has any foundation? It certainly fits in quite well with many known facts, though some of the epidemiological data are hard to reconcile with this – or indeed any other – physiological theory. First, it is obvious that the cause of SIDS is a multi-factorial. In other words, a number of factors have to act on a given baby at a given time in order to cause death. Using the PSA theory, there must first be a baby with an inborn tendency to PSA: it is likely that certain factors such as prematurity and low birth-weight may be related to the late development of the stability of the breathing mechanism. Second, there is very frequently some kind of virus infection in these infants which explains the presence of the virus throughout the tissues and perhaps some narrowing of the breathing passages. There may also be some other factors such as abnormality and insensitivity of the chemical receptors for oxygen or carbon dioxide. If all these factors are present in one infant, then there would appear to be a substantial risk of SIDS occurring.

There is a considerable amount of direct pathological and physiological evidence that hypoxia (deficiency of oxygen) and perhaps an abnormality of the chemical receptors does exist in some infants. Much of the work has been done in the United States where Richard Naeye has reported the following features:

1. The walls of the pulmonary arteries in the lung are thicker than in non-SIDS infants. This is a sign of long-standing oxygen lack in the body.

2. A different type of fat, called 'brown fat', tends to remain around the adrenal glands.

3. The right ventricle of the heart may be enlarged, related to the thickening of the pulmonary arteries.

4. Red blood cells may be formed in the liver as a response to increased need for added production which cannot be coped with in the usual way in the bone marrow.

5. There may be abnormalities in the fine structure of the carotid body, the microscopic collection of nerve endings on the large arteries in the neck, which are responsible for monitoring the oxygen content of the arterial blood.

6. The medulla or central part of the suprarenal glands on top of the kidneys, which produce adrenaline, may show an increase in 'chromaffin tissue', another marker of hypoxia.

7. The brain tissue, especially in the brainstem and central areas, may show 'gliosis', a replacement of the normal nervous tissue by a more inert type of supporting fibre, especially in the region of the respiratory centres. Other workers apart from Naeye have described this change.

It must be said that other researchers have failed to confirm all of Richard Naeye's findings, but there is substantial evidence to show that a state of chronic, i.e. long-standing, oxygen lack does occur in many SIDS victims, if sufficiently refined methods of investigation are used. For instance, the well-known Sheffield research team led by Professor John Emery, have found that there was a fatty replacement on a microscopic scale in parts of the brainstem, which they attribute to chronic hypoxia.

Many other medical workers have investigated problems connected with the central theme of hypoxia and sleep apnoea – in fact, this aspect now dominates most scientific meetings concerned with sudden infant death and the medical journals carry a stream of research articles describing new findings of one sort or another. The prime researcher in this field is Dr Alfred Steinschneider of New York, who first put forward this theory in 1972 and has been working energetically on it ever since. He is now engaged on a very large prospective survey (looking ahead, rather than backward) of about 1000 infants each year, to evaluate the incidence and degree of sleep apnoea.

Other factors which may well contribute to the hypoxia have been investigated, many of the research schemes still being pursued. One concerns the posture of the head. Many SIDS babies are thought to be somewhat hypotonic, that is, they have slack muscles and poor muscle tone throughout the body, especially in the neck, which has to support the relatively larger head of an infant. This sagging of the head may worsen the efficiency of the air passages at mouth and neck level, especially during sleep and feeding. The narrowing of the upper parts of the respiratory passages – the nose, mouth and throat – is called obstructive apnoea, as opposed to the central apnoea of weak drive delivered from the respiratory centres in the brainstem. Obstructive apnoea is a more potent producer of hypoxia than central apnoea, as it mechanically stops the inflow of air, but the two processes may combine on an intermittent basis to render the infant chronically short of oxygen over a period of months, which then leads to the set of pathological signs found by Richard Naeye.

An Australian specialist, Doctor Tonkin, thinks that the airway may sometimes be blocked at the level of the palate, at the back of the throat, especially during sleep and when strongly sucking. Other researchers have followed up this idea and suggested that flexion – the bending forward – of the neck may also block the airway. They found two infants in whom apnoea was produced when this posture was taken up. A large muscular tongue and a sucking action can collapse the soft walls of the back of the throat; they think that the walls of the throat come together on breathing in, rather like sucking hard on a wet drinking-straw, which then flattens and fails to pass any liquid.

These ideas are not, of course, thought to be the actual cause of any individual cot death, but are mechanisms which may occur sporadically and perhaps frequently during the first few months of a baby's life, leading to the long-term hypoxia which may cause the infant to develop an unstable heart condition. Periods of bradycardia (slow heart beat) are common in hypoxia and on one particular occasion, with perhaps an intense period of hypoxia, the infant may get into an Ondine's Curse situation, with entry to the fatal descending spiral of hypoxia – apnoea – bradycardia – worse hypoxia – heart failure cycle which leads to death unless interrupted. Of course, many infants climb out of the spiral, or some interruption may break the pattern. These cases may never then be recognised, because thankfully they are back to normal next morning and the lucky parents unaware that anything had been wrong. Probably the majority of such events in some of the 500–700 babes fortunately end in nothing. A few are recognised, but the infants do not die, these being the near-misses which we shall discuss shortly.

A great deal of research is now going into the study of various types of airway obstruction. The relative roles of nasal narrowing, closure of the glottis (entrance to the voice box) and closure of the vocal cords are being investigated. The research aspects are in part passing from the pathologist into the more academic realms of the respiratory physiologist and the anatomist, who study the air passages and their functions.

While still on the subject of airway narrowing, one further possibility must be mentioned. Off and on for a number of years, the possibility of airway obstruction at laryngeal level has been considered. The larynx is the voice box or Adam's apple in the throat, which carries the vocal cords, between which all our breathing air has to pass. If the cords are tightly shut, as in the first stages of a cough, then obviously no air can enter or leave. It was suggested a long time ago that a supposed condition called laryngeal spasm might cause SIDS by merely cutting off the air – this was supposedly given credence in those days when the little petechial haemorrhages on the lungs and thymus were thought to be due to pure obstructive apnoea . . . a view which in some ways has been revived by those who think that they are due to the infant's trying to breathe against a closed glottis (the entrance to the larynx). This spasm of the larynx can be caused by tetany, a defect in the calcium content of the blood which makes muscles very irritable and prone to spasm. We touched on this earlier in our list of theories, but showed that the calcium idea was found to be a non-starter. Some evidence of rickets has also been found, primarily by a professor in Austria, but though rib changes sometimes suggest a sub-clinical calcium defect, no real proof has been forthcoming to substantiate the vocal cord/calcium spasm theory.

The laryngeal hypothesis has some other facts in its favour in that the edges of the vocal cords are frequently found to be damaged, when examined microscopically, as if they had been rubbing together or forcibly pushed together. Another more recent theory would help to link with sleep apnoea and hypoxia. To follow this one we have to recall that two of Naeye's signs of chronic oxygen lack were thickened pulmonary arteries in the lungs and an enlarged right ventricle in the heart. Now one of the nerves which supplies and controls the vocal cords – the recurrent laryngeal on the left side – passes from the neck, deeply into the chest and hooks round the remains of the ductus arteriosus (the connecting channel that by-passes the lungs in fetal life).

This left recurrent laryngeal nerve, according to Dr Vessilinova-Jenkins, may be trapped at the point where it hooks round the ductus connecting the aorta to the pulmonary artery, because of the swelling of the pulmonary artery caused by high pulmonary pressure, in turn caused by hypoxia affecting the pulmonary arteries, as described by Dr Naeye. This entrapment causes damage to the nerve fibres and partly paralyses the left vocal cord, which then sags into the mid-line of the larynx, reducing the already poor airway. It is well known to ear, nose and throat surgeons that the left vocal cord is often weak in infants and less brisk in its movements than the right. Dr Jenkins has included this nerve defect in the whole complex system of sleep apnoea and hypoxia that seems to be emerging out of so much diverse research.

Yet another claim in this area is that the other nerves which supply the vocal cords, the superior laryngeal nerves, may be affected by regurgitation of stomach contents into the upper part of the gullet, the so-called gastro-oesophageal reflex.

Figure 13 summarises some of these suggested factors of SIDS.

The topic of sleep apnoea will be discussed again when we look at possible ways of preventing SIDS, for at the present time, detection and warning of dangerous sleep apnoea seems the most profitable avenue of trying to deal with the tragic syndrome – though even at this stage it must be said that some very expert child health specialists warn that they have considerable reservations about getting too enthusiastic and hopeful.

The near-miss SIDS infant

One of the most important and scientifically interesting developments in the whole area of sudden infant death study in recent years has been the appreciation of near-miss babies. In a syndrome which previously was investigatable only by backward-looking post-mortem examinations, it was a major step forward to have even limited material to examine in the live state.

Increasingly in these recent years, going back less than a decade, it has been recognised that a small proportion of cot deaths were preceded by incidents which were obviously a near-miss on a previous occasion. Following this, the same

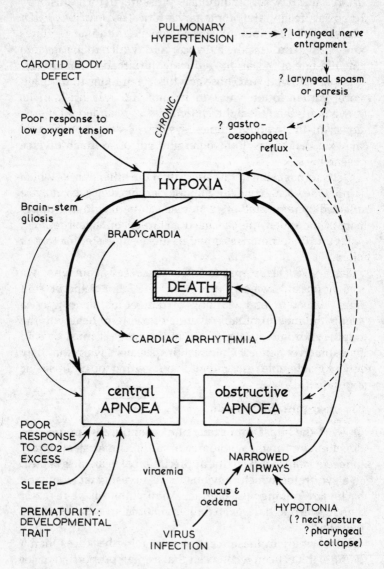

Fig. 13 A complex mechanism – some of the suggested factors in SIDS

kind of near tragedy has been detected in other infants who happily survived to reach the virtually safe age of eight to ten months.

According to present usage, a definition of a near-miss SIDS is a baby who has ceased breathing and who seems to have died suddenly and unexpectedly, but whose life was saved by timely intervention. The intervention need not be any sophisticated medical procedure such as the kiss of life or external cardiac massage, though these have been used – quite often, it was merely the mother's scooping up the baby in a panic and rushing off to the nearest neighbour, doctor or accident department of her local hospital.

Some mothers had reported, when giving the circumstances of their baby's death, that the child had had some kind of episode days or even weeks before. The description varied from 'having a funny turn' to a detailed picture of what had happened. A frequent story was of the mother's having passed the child's cot, sometimes quite casually, and unexpectedly seeing it either to be pale and apparently lifeless or sometimes blue in the face or at the lips. Naturally aghast and panic-stricken, the mother would snatch up the child and either try to revive it herself or rush off with it to get assistance. In fact, this was the same pattern as in many true SIDS, but in these near-misses, the babe revived, often rapidly and spontaneously, due to the stimulation of being vigorously moved, which presumably broke the vicious circle of apnoea and hypoxia before it had descended to irretrievable heart arrest. Others had to be hurried to a doctor or hospital, where urgent resuscitation was carried out with success. This sometimes took place in an ambulance, where an experienced crew-man used his expertise and experience together with emergency oxygen.

Regrettably, a few fell between the actual cot death condition and complete recovery; the re-starting of respiration and heart beat had been delayed those few moments too long, so that irreparable brain damage occurred from oxygen lack. Brain death was the inevitable outcome eventually because the interval between the onset of hypoxia and the revival was too long to save the oxygen-sensitive brain tissue.

The babes which survived their near-misses were usually normal to general examination and most went on to become normal, healthy children, passing the danger threshold for SIDS and merging into the healthy population. However, when tested by more sensitive and sophisticated methods, it became apparent that many near-misses were by no means totally normal or healthy until they graduated into an older age bracket. Indeed, some regrettably died a cot death a short time later, which is how the group became recognised. These days, a near-miss is known to be in a vulnerable state for a number of months and is therefore watched very carefully and usually monitored under close supervision to prevent, if at all possible, the predisposing factors from striking again.

The fact that the snatching up of the child often returned the baby to normal has been used as additional evidence that the mode of death is a deepening cardiorespiratory depression, which can be interrupted by any physical stimulation such as the handling of the child during panic or, where the spiral has become more deeply entrenched, by resuscitatory measures.

Further study of near-miss babies has revealed that a wide spectrum of abnormalities is often present. For example, in 1976, 12 near-miss infants were studied at Stanford University in the United States. They were continuously monitored for 24 hours, to study their sleep state and their heart and lung functions. These were then compared with similar investigations on seven other babies who were known to be low risk for SIDS and who had never had any unusual episodes. The near-misses much more often showed periods of sleep apnoea, both from central failure of respiratory control by the brain and from obstruction of the air passages.

Associated with these episodes was marked bradycardia (slowing of the heart rate), which sometimes also occurred even when the breathing pattern seemed normal. One child actually went into asystole (heart stoppage) during one of these runs of slow heart rate. Both these functions of breathing and heart rate are related to the autonomic nervous system and it seems almost certain that SIDS babies and potential cot deaths have some malfunction of this automatic part of the central nervous system which controls our internal machinery.

One baby girl being studied at Stanford actually died at 21 weeks of age, after being studied because of a near-miss at about 14 weeks. Study of the data on breathing patterns in this child showed there had been numerous episodes of central and obstructive apnoea compared with other control infants. Abnormalities in the brainstem, especially in and around the autonomic control nuclei in the brainstem, were found by sophisticated techniques; these resembled the gliosis described by Naeye and other workers.

Other studies elsewhere on near-miss babies have amply confirmed that there are abnormalities in the heart function, especially as recorded by ECG (electrocardiograms). Part of the ECG tracing (the Q-T interval) was found to be significantly shorter during sleep, than control infants. Many other studies on heart and respiratory function in near-miss children have been published and most confirm some abnormality, worse in sleep and worsened by any reduction in the oxygen supply to the lungs.

Dr Marie Valdes-Dapena, the indefatigable analyst of the huge medical literature on SIDS, sums it up by saying: 'Thus it can be said with some degree of assurance, that near-miss infants are different from normal infants, not only in regard to physiologic functions, especially cardiac and respiratory, but also that they are at special risk for sudden death, a fact that was earlier suspected, but has now been established.'

4 · After the tragedy

Although very energetic research is now going on in a number of countries, in the present state of medical knowledge there is unfortunately no way of preventing the sudden infant death syndrome – though, as will be described in a later chapter, some tentative measures are in the experimental stage. Until such time as we have reliable preventive methods, every effort has to be made to comfort and support the bereaved parents. Certainly, nothing should be done by anyone which actually worsens their situation.

A number of defects in the medical, legal and administrative handling of afflicted parents have been only too apparent in the past – and, regrettably, a number survive today. When a SIDS tragedy occurs, the parents are shocked, bewildered and above all suspicious that they themselves are somehow partly to blame. Though this last aspect mainly affects the mother, the whole sad affair has a much greater impact on the father than is generally realised, mainly due to conventional notions that the male has to keep a stiff upper lip and suppress his emotions in order to be more supportive to his wife. Probably the father has received relatively scant attention from counsellors in the past, though it is inevitable that the mother should receive the major part of the sympathy and support.

She almost always feels self-recrimination, whether she recognises it or not. The feelings of guilt may be so obvious that a frank anxiety state may develop and the author is aware of at least two instances where the mother actually committed suicide. Expression of a wish to die, especially 'to join my baby' are not all that uncommon, though thankfully they are usually transitory – here again, the need for prompt and effective counselling and, in extreme cases, psychiatric help is demonstrated.

In most cases the mother has a nagging feeling that somehow, something she did or something she failed to do was the cause of, or a contribution to, her baby's death. Prolonged reassurance and explanation often fail to remove the obstinate convictions, even against all logic, and time alone is likely to alleviate this nagging self-reproach.

Because of the often unsatisfactory and uncertain explanations given – which sometimes amount to apparent evasiveness – the parents may constantly search for a rational explanation of this sudden catastrophe that has descended on their family like a thunderbolt. Although intensely sad, other types of infant death such as cancers, leukaemia and congenital defects may be easier for parents to bear than the lightning stroke of SIDS.

First, these other diseases are known about beforehand and death is not unexpected, so that, tragic though it be, the parents have had some time to begin adjusting to and anticipating the fatal outcome. In addition, these types of disease invariably have a definite medical diagnosis attached to them, so the parents know when the child is very ill – and when it eventually dies – that the malignant disease or congenital defect was something that was not treatable or avoidable. It has a definite medical label, recognised by doctors, who could explain before and after the death the nature and inevitability of the illness.

In SIDS, all this is lacking. The child is either quite healthy or has trivial symptoms – then the next day it is dead. The doctors cannot put a true cause to the death, even after a post-mortem examination. Sometimes the doctor seems equally bewildered, evasive or just plain ignorant of the condition. Unless efficient and authoritative counselling is available, a question-mark continues to hang over the death, not least in the minds of the parents. This may last for the rest of their lives and often persists in an acute form for many months. The author has met several older parents who lost a child from SIDS many years earlier and yet they told him that they still had nagging doubts about the cause of death and wondered still whether or not they had in some way contributed to it.

The troubles of the bereaved parents may be accentuated from several different directions, especially where there is little or no awareness on the part of supportive services – such a situation was almost universal a decade or two ago. The following factors are those which have an adverse effect, often of drastic proportions, upon the mental and even physical welfare of the parents:

The family physician

Though matters have improved considerably in the past few years – mainly because of publicity about the sudden infant death syndrome and the efforts of organisations such as The Foundation for the Study of Infant Deaths – the medical profession cannot feel proud of its record in former years as a supportive element in SIDS. The family physician often played too small a role in this family tragedy and was often obviously reluctant to become too involved, a situation which still exists today.

When a cot death occurs, the frantic parent usually rushes with the child either to a hospital or calls her own family doctor to the home. Unfortunately, this latter contact may all too frequently be the only part which the general practitioner plays in the drama, his participation being virtually only as a certifier of death. Though thankfully, the situation is improving rapidly, many SIDS parents bitterly relate a similar story about their medical adviser. The doctor may come to the house, examine the baby, declare it to be dead and then vanish never to be seen again. A number of parents have reported that their doctor seemed deliberately to avoid them in the future, possibly because he felt inadequate in being unable to counsel them.

Certainly in past years, few general practitioners knew much, if anything, about cot death. They had no answers for the many questions posed by the parents and felt professionally embarrassed at their own lack of ability. This was – and often still is – a defect in the training of many doctors, who rarely hear anything of the sudden infant death syndrome in their medical schools. Hopefully, the almost explosive increase in research and publications in the past few years has generated a new interest among professional people but this will take some time to percolate into teaching programmes. Even now, when SIDS has become a prominent matter for research and discussion, few medical schools find a place for it in their crowded curriculum. Paediatricians are not all that familiar with the syndrome because it rarely occurs in hospital. General pathologists rarely see cases, except those with an appreciable stake in coroner's work. It is the forensic pathologist, a very rare species these days, who has the only academic contact both with SIDS and medical students. Even this confluence has declined to insignificance, especially in British medical schools, so there is little opportunity for general practitioners to gain any exposure to this subject during training. Those GPs who qualified some years ago will certainly have had no instruction as students on the matter and will only have heard of SIDS through perhaps some sporadic postgraduate lecture and in the hard school of clinical experience. However, as the average family doctor will only see two or three cases in his professional life, the opportunities to learn are sparse and the unfortunate families who provide this meagre experience have no opportunity to benefit.

This is not much excuse for the general supportive counselling which a doctor should be able to supply, even if he has no way of being completely *au fait* with current trends in SIDS research. Though he may know little about recent advances in the topic, his general medical training and his professional acumen and bedside manner should surely offer some comfort to the parents – and he should be able to direct them to a source of more specialised counselling.

It is a matter of regret that so many of the parents questioned in the Foundation survey reported such a deficiency in the family practitioner's ability to provide help and solace.

Another defect which sometimes occurs is that the family doctor does not even know that the tragedy has taken place. Where, as quite often happens, the babe is rushed to a hospital and is certified dead there, no one gets around to telling the GP. Although theoretically the coroner's investigation should refer back to him for a clinical history, quite often the hospital doctor reports the death and the general practitioner is left in ignorance. On some dreadful occasions, the GP has actually turned up at the house days later to make some routine call on the baby, who might have been seen when it had the slight premonitory symptoms a week or so earlier. It can be a major public relations disaster, as far as both doctor and family are concerned, for a doctor to call and find his small patient gone, with a grieving family shocked by his ignorance.

Parents are often dissatisfied with their general practitioner and in one series of SIDS investigated no less than one-third of all parents changed their doctor after the event, having apparently lost faith in his abilities. Though this was often unfounded and perhaps quite unfair, it reflects the uneasy situation that one hopes is becoming much less common. In retrospective enquiries from parents, the most frequent complaints included the fact that the doctor never returned after the first urgent visit, never later enquired after their welfare and never appeared to be aware of or made any enquiries about the outcome of the post-mortem or returned to try to explain the results when they were available.

This rather harsh commentary must be balanced by mention of those doctors whose conduct was exemplary and whose support of the parents in this difficult time was the greatest factor in their recovery process. Many general practitioners – especially the younger ones – do all in their power to explain the nature of SIDS, though in the present state of knowledge and teaching this might be slight enough. They return soon after the death – the same day – to enquire after the welfare of the parents and perhaps to prescribe some sedative. Some caution should be exercised here: it has been shown that heavy sedation may be counter-productive if it is a barrier to the normal process of bereavement and grieving. The tragedy has to be endured, suffered and eventually rationalised and to retard this unduly by knocking out the mother with drugs may prolong or distort the process. The experienced doctor will know how to fit his actions to the needs of individual cases.

Mention has already been made of the need for the doctor to return frequently in the first few days to explain the legal and administrative processes such as the coroner's enquiry and to interpret the post-mortem findings. There might later be more practical advice needed, such as information on re-housing and explanations about the apparent length and intractability of the feelings of reproach and grief. They should make themselves available for further counselling over a long period and give advice where needed about the reactions of other children in the family, as well as advice about having a new baby.

The Foundation for the Study of Infant Deaths have issued a check list for general practitioners, as part of their excellent series of short leaflets on several aspects of sudden infant death. The text reads as follows:

Check List

*Unexpected Infant Death – Cot Death –
GP Support of the Family*

One baby in every 500 live births dies unexpectedly for no obvious reason between the ages of 1 week and 2 years, 90% before 8 months. Although such tragedies are comparatively rare, in a group practice of 2 or 3 doctors, a cot death is likely to occur every 3 to 5 years.

A GP may be called to the home or the baby rushed to the surgery; often the baby is taken directly to a hospital casualty department. GPs should ensure in advance that coroners, hospitals and medical deputising services would inform the family doctor immediately of an unexpected infant death.

The following notes are intended to help doctors managing a cot death for the first time.

1. As soon as you hear of the baby's death, *contact the family* to

express sympathy, by a home visit if possible. Early support prevents later misunderstandings.

2. Unless there is an obvious injury, a history of illness or the parental attitude arouses suspicion, tell the parents it appears to be a cot death but that a post-mortem examination will be necessary to establish the cause of death. If death remains unexplained, it may be registered as 'sudden infant death syndrome'. Some parents want to see or hold their child after death is confirmed but before the body is taken to the mortuary.

3. Explain the *coroner's duty*, the possibility of an inquest and warn parents that they may be required to identify the body. Advise the parents that they will be asked to make a statement to the coroner's officer or police and that bedding may be taken for examination to help establish the cause of death. If necessary, give advice on registering the death and making funeral arrangements. Coroner's officer may need to know the parents' choice of burial or cremation.

4. If considering offering parents a drug to alleviate the initial shock, it is known that many do not want anxiolytics or anti-depressants, but prefer something to induce sleep.

5. If the mother was breast feeding, give advice on suppression of lactation; prescribe medication and advise her to leave the breasts alone except to empty them once a day if an easy method is available.

6. Take particular note of *siblings*. Remember that twin babies carry extra risk of cot death and that a surviving twin may need hospitalisation for observation. Give guidance on the emotional needs of siblings, who may be neglected or overprotected; reassure parents that older children are not at risk.

7. Advise parents of likely *grief reactions* such as aching arms, hearing the baby cry, distressing dreams and strong positive or negative sexual feelings, but reassure them that these and other symptoms such as loss of appetite and sleeplessness are normal and temporary. Anger, sometimes directed toward the GP, guilt and self-blame, especially on the part of the mother, are common grief reactions for which the doctor should be prepared.

8. Offer parents copies of the leaflet *'Information for Parents Following the Sudden and Unexpected Death of their Baby'*, and the address of the *Foundation*. In addition to sponsoring medical research, the Foundation offers further support and information and can put parents in touch with others who have previously suffered a similar bereavement.

9. Make sure that parents have a relative or close friend very near them during the 48 hours after the death and offer explanation to them and to the minister of religion. Make sure the family's *health visitor* and other members of the primary health care team know of the baby's death and are prepared to give continued support.

10. Arrange a subsequent meeting with parents to discuss the cause of death. Make sure the coroner informs you of the initial and final post-mortem findings and consult with the pathologist if any clarification is needed.

11. Offer parents a later interview with a paediatrician both for themselves and the siblings. An independent opinion is mutually beneficial to the parents and the GP restoring parental confidence in the primary care team and sharing some of the load of counselling, particularly concerning future children.

12. Parents who have lost a baby unexpectedly will need extra care and support with their subsequent children from their obstetrician, paediatrician, general practitioner and health visitor.

The hospital

Many infant victims of SIDS are taken immediately to hospital accident and emergency departments, usually by the parents' rushing them there in their own or a neighbour's car or by calling the ambulance service. This by-passes their general practitioner, but may be the best course where the GP is out on domiciliary visits and cannot be immediately contacted. On arrival at such a casualty department, the infant is seen and certified dead, either immediately or after attempted resuscitation.

Though the purely medical aspects rarely give rise to any criticism later, the subsequent handling of the tragedy may leave much to be desired. This became very evident from the replies to the Foundation survey from parents who had suffered a SIDS in their family. There were many complaints about the way in which the family was handled by hospitals, albeit without any intention to hurt or obstruct.

Accident and emergency departments are invariably overworked and often frantically busy, but in such a profoundly tragic situation as a sudden infant death, even this should not be an excuse for not following a humane and sympathetic code of practice. The doctor who certifies death may be relatively junior, especially in smaller hospitals and at night or early morning. Like many family doctors, he may know little or nothing about SIDS and quite often has never had to deal with a case before.

The doctor, after attempted revival and then his professional duty of confirming death, may vanish after a few relatively perfunctory words of sympathy. He may gladly pass the more social responsibilities over to the casualty sister or staff nurse and slip away to his many other duties. Many families record that they had little or no explanation from the doctor and may even have been viewed with some suspicion because of the misplaced overspill of publicity about child abuse – the 'battered baby', with which sudden infant death is not infrequently confused.

The hospital doctor may even have seen the baby in the ambulance outside the casualty department; having been examined and pronounced dead, it may then even be driven direct to the mortuary without ever entering the hospital. This practice is to be condemned and even if the ambulance crew are satisfied that the baby is probably dead on arrival, the examination should be carried out in the relatively decent privacy of an examination room or cubicle and not a perfunctory glance be given in the dim light of an ambulance interior, sometimes with the aid of a torch.

The hospital doctor, like the GP, has no option but to refer the death for medico-legal investigation, i.e. report to the coroner, procurator, medical examiner, etc, depending upon the geographical circumstances. Once this is done, many hospital casualty departments seem to clamp a legal Iron Curtain around the infant body, under some misapprehension that a medico-legal case has some affinities with Sherlock Holmes and the preservation of clues.

It is true that precautions must be taken with other deaths, either child or adult, where frankly criminal or suspicious circumstances exist, but in the relatively common and well-recognised sudden infant death syndrome, this is unnecessary.

Many parents have said that once declared dead, the baby's body was immediately taken away from them or they were hustled out of the examination room. The body was then taken to the mortuary and they were expressly forbidden to go near it or touch it 'because it was now a police case'.

Here we see a prime psychological mistake, in that the rapid and abrupt separation of the mother and father from the deceased infant can lead to a most profound increase in intensity and duration of grieving. Many mothers—and indeed fathers—wish to touch or hold their child for the last time, to 'say goodbye' to it and perhaps require this final contact in order to realise that it is indeed irrevocably dead. This is not uncommonly deprived them in some hospitals, usually by a senior nurse or sister, who has an erroneous and misplaced idea of her public duty in relation to the coroner's investigation.

This attitude may be perpetuated in the hospital mortuary. Usually the body has to be formally identified at a later time and it may be done in the mortuary chapel, but many such places are a funereal chamber complete with glass partition and forbidding velvet curtains. The parents may be confined behind the screen, being made to view the child at a distance in a dimly lit chamber redolent of mysterious and inimical rites. Many parents have said that mortuary staff have forbidden them to approach or handle the body 'because it is a coroner's case'. This attitude is desperately wrong, but thankfully it has been recognised widely in recent years and many enlightened hospitals have made strenuous efforts to lighten the burden placed on the already desperately grieving parents.

One such centre is Sheffield, so well known for its work in the scientific and epidemiological aspects of SIDS. In large measure due to the efforts of Professor John Emery and his colleagues, much attention is paid to the psychological welfare of the parents, as well as to the scientific research.

A recent article from the Children's Hospital in Sheffield describes how the arrival of a dead child – from any cause – is treated as a medical emergency. At night, a senior nurse deals with the parents and passes them on to the mortuary technician in the morning. In the daytime, this technician, a woman of mature years and experience and herself a grandmother, organises most aspects of the death procedure and acts as the initial friend and counsellor of the parents. Explanations and advice on funeral arrangements, supply of counselling leaflets, etc., are provided by the technician, who liaises with the medical and coroner's staff on behalf of the parents.

The mother and father are encouraged to see and cuddle the child if they so wish and the technician makes sure that the body is as presentable as possible, both before and after a post-mortem. Before the baby leaves the mortuary, the technician dresses it according to the preference of the parents and, if necessary, uses make-up judiciously to restore it to the best possible appearance. She may add a favourite cuddly toy and again the parents are quite welcome to spend as long as they wish in a final farewell – a far cry from the authoritarian abruptness of some institutions.

The Foundation for the Study of Infant Deaths has issued a card for hospital casualty departments, which suggests a practical code of behaviour in this situation and can be displayed in the staff area of the department to alert doctors and nurses about the urgency and importance of proper handling of a sudden infant death. The text reads:

Unexpected Infant Deaths
Guidelines for Accident and Emergency Departments
Cot Death – Sudden Infant Death Syndrome (SIDS)

One baby in every 500 live births dies suddenly and unexpectedly between the ages of 1 week and 2 years. There are about 2000 of these deaths a year in the United Kingdom, accounting for half the deaths in this age group. Babies die unexpectedly for many reasons, in some cases the cause of death is evident at post-mortem examination. This may for example reveal evidence of an unsuspected abnormality or of a severe illness such as meningitis or pneumonia. In the majority, however, the cause is obscure and these are called cot deaths or the sudden infant death syndrome. Post-mortem evidence of minor infection which probably contributed to death is sometimes found and may be mentioned as the registered cause of death with SIDS or unexpected death in infancy as an associated cause. In others, nothing significant is found. Sudden infant death syndrome is now accepted internationally as a natural registrable cause of death.

In a typical case, an apparently normal baby, whose symptoms of illness, if any, appear trivial is put to rest; a few minutes or hours later the infant is found dead. Cot deaths are more common in the winter months, amongst boys and amongst babies of low birth weight; there is a peak incidence at 2–5 months of age and most deaths appear to occur during sleep.

Parents' reactions and fears

Shocked and distraught, the parents often fear that they in some way were responsible and search through all they did or did not do for a reason for the death. Such guilt feelings are a normal reaction, but quite unfounded.

Sometimes the baby is found face down with the bedclothes over him and the parents are frightened that the infant suffocated; many babies normally sleep like that with no harmful effects.

Occasionally vomit, which may be tinged with blood, is found around the mouth or on the bedding; this usually occurs during or after death and is seldom the cause of death.

Sometimes a relative or babysitter is looking after the baby when he dies. It is important that everyone understands that SIDS is a well recognised, though little understood condition and that blame is attached to no one.

Sequence of Action in Accident and Emergency Department

1. Verification of death should be made in the Accident Department, rather than in the ambulance.
2. If resuscitation is attempted or while the baby's condition is being evaluated, a brief history of the baby's health and recent events should be taken from an accompanying parent.
3. Every effort should be made to provide a room or privacy for the distressed parents.
4. Ensure that a suitable person is looking after the baby's brothers and sisters who may have come with the parent.
5. If only one parent is present and agrees, contact the other parent or relatives.
6. INFORM (i) a member of the paediatric department.
7. INFORM (ii) hospital chaplain if parents request that a dying child is to be baptised or wish for his support.
8. Review information briefly before breaking the news that the baby is dead. Parents will need privacy in which to express their grief.
9. After an appropriate interval, inform parents of the need for a post-mortem examination to establish the cause of death, which will be arranged by the coroner.
10. Unless there is a history of diagnosed illness, obvious signs of injury or the parental attitude arouses suspicion, explain to the parents that the death appears to be a cot death (also called sudden death in infancy syndrome).
11. Explain to parents that it is the coroner's duty to investigate all sudden deaths of unknown cause and that they will be asked to make a statement to the coroner's officer or police, who may visit their home and may take the baby's bedding for examination to establish the cause of death. This does not mean that anyone will be blamed or that an inquest will necessarily be held.
12. INFORM (iii) hospital social work department. Someone should remain with the parents until they leave.
13. INFORM (iv) coroner's officer and explain whether the death appears to be natural or unnatural.

14. Offer the parents the opportunity to see their baby and let them hold him before he is taken to the mortuary. The infant should be clothed and made as presentable as possible.

15. If identification of the body to the coroner's officer or police is required, a member of staff or the hospital chaplain should accompany the parents to the mortuary.

16. Offer parents copies of the leaflet *Information for Parents Following the Sudden and Unexpected Death of Their Baby* which gives the address and telephone number of the Foundation for the Study of Infant Deaths.

17. Discuss with parents arrangements for continued support.

18. INFORM (v) the family doctor
                (vi) the health visitor
                (vii) social worker if already involved with family.

19. The mother, if breast feeding, will need immediate advice on the suppression of lactation.

20. Ensure that the parents have suitable transport to take them home.

Later support

It is important for a doctor to explain to the parents as soon as possible the initial post-mortem findings and the registered cause of death, preferably after consulting with the pathologist. It is helpful for a paediatrician to undertake this and he will need to inform the GP. Alternatively, the family doctor may wish to do so. A paediatric consultation is often helpful a few weeks later if the parents then wish to ask further questions or if further detailed post-mortem studies clarify the cause of death.

The paediatrician

As mentioned in the last paragraph of the leaflet, it is often helpful to have an interview at some stage with a consultant paediatrician, a specialist in child health from the local hospital or medical centre.

It must be said that until a couple of decades ago, paediatricians shared in the general ignorance of doctors about cot death. They rarely came into contact with SIDS, as these rarely occur in hospital wards. This is because only a relatively small fraction of the total child population is in hospital at any one time, so the 1 in 500 ratio at about the danger period of two to four months is only going to put a very small number of hospitalised babies at risk. In addition, wards are busy places, with alert nurses bustling about, even at the early hour when most SIDS occur and any infant who might be sinking into an apnoeic state may well be seen and stimulated or revived. In fact, a number of the near-miss cases described elsewhere in this book, have been picked up in hospitals, especially in intensive care units which contain a selected population including a higher proportion of at-risk children. As cot deaths almost all died at home or in casualty departments, paediatricians had little opportunity to familiarise themselves with the syndrome; however, this slow start has been more than made up for during the sudden arousal of interest since about 1960. The medical journals have been frequently publishing articles on SIDS, both in general journals and in pathology, forensic medicine, epidemiology and paediatric periodicals.

Paediatricians are now fully conversant with the syndrome and its problems for the family and can provide a potent back-up in counselling, especially where the parents would like an independent opinion. This often helps to restore their confidence in their own family doctor, as the paediatrician can explain that the GP's apparent inability to have foreseen or prevented the tragedy was quite unavoidable, in that no other doctor could have done anything different. The paediatrician can also be very valuable in reassuring parents about the low risk in subsequent births. Where an unusually high degree of apprehension exists, he might be able to arrange for early monitoring of a new baby, perhaps with the co-operation of the obstetrician.

An interview with a specialist in child health is probably most fruitful after the acute phase of bereavement is over. Some parents may also like to talk to the pathologist who carried out the post-mortem examination and again this is best done after an interval in which the more emotive phase has subsided. Some pathologists are reluctant to get involved with parents, even sheltering behind the façade of the coroner's procedure, claiming that they cannot discuss a legal examination. This is not really realistic and may in some cases be related to the fact that some doctors choose pathology because it is a non-clinical speciality in which they do not have much, if any, contact with patients. Dr Lester Adelson of the United States has pointed out in an excellent publication the forensic pathologist is a 'physician to the bereaved' and that a sympathetic explanation of what the post-mortem revealed can go a long way towards resolving and dispelling doubts and sometimes bizarre misapprehensions which the relatives may have about the death.

The police

Next in our survey of those involved in the aftermath of a sudden infant death, come the police. As virtually all SIDS become the subject of a medico-legal investigation, whatever the geographical variation in the style of enquiry, some agency has to search after the facts. In Britain, this is either the coroner's officer or the police – the former often being plain-clothes police officers. In a medical examiner system, the investigating officers from the ME's Office will make these enquiries.

It is a matter for local practice whether the enquiries are made at the home of the family or whether the parents are required to attend at the office of the investigators. In Britain, local variations occur but it is common practice for a uniformed police officer to visit the house to obtain a history of the circumstances surrounding the child's death. This is usually done on the day of the death or day following.

Where the investigating officer is a regular coroner's officer, well used to this type of work and used to interviewing recently bereaved people, then the situation may be fairly satisfactory. He may or may not be a uniformed officer, but where a duty constable visits the house the appearance of obvious police interest and activity in the matter is undesirable. The neighbours frequently misinterpret this as evidence of some suspicious circumstance, on the 'where there's smoke, there's fire' principle. Public confusion

of SIDS with the even more publicised child abuse syndrome
has led to considerable unpleasantness in the past, especially
where a later injudicious remark by a neighbour or even
relative about the presence of the police triggers resentment
in the ultra-sensitive mother or father.

The parents themselves may well be upset by the
appearance of the police at their door and may be even more
offended if he insists on carrying off bedding and pillows in
full view of the neighbours peering from behind their
curtains. The practice of taking cot, mattress and bedding for
some spurious examination is an anachronistic hangover
from the lingering conviction that SIDS is somehow related to
overlaying and suffocation. In the current state of medical
thinking about the patho-physiology of SIDS, any examination of bedding is futile – and who really wants to examine it?
The pathologist who knows anything about SIDS will gain
nothing by finding a little dried nasal or pulmonary oedema
fluid on a pillow; the significance of vomit in the actual air
passages is obscure, so vomit on a blanket which probably
got there during agonal regurgitation is even less help.

Returning to the police role, where the officer is not a
regular coroner's officer, he might well be totally unaware of
the existence of the sudden infant death syndrome and
conduct a heavy-handed interrogation completely misdirected towards confirming or excluding child abuse,
deliberate suffocation or, at best, accidental asphyxia.
Bereaved parents have reported, in surveys made of the
administrative procedures following a cot death, that some
police officers were frankly hostile or suspicious. The effect of
this upon a bewildered, self-reproachful and acutely grieving
young mother a few hours after losing her child can well be
imagined.

Thankfully, these troubles have decreased, mainly because
of the activities of organisations who have approached the
coroners, but all black spots have not yet been eradicated.

It has been recommended – and is in fact the practice in
some areas – that no home visits are made by the police,
especially by uniformed officers. Interviews are conducted at

the police station or coroner's office, though sometimes the emotional and physical state of the mother may make this impracticable. The father may often provide sufficient information in this instance. In other regions, use is made of plain-clothes women police officers with the obvious merit of a more sympathetic rapport between a woman and a mother.

Whatever the local practice, sympathy, tact and at least some knowledge of the nature of SIDS is a prerequisite for the investigator. Wherever possible, some other person with a sound knowledge of cot death, such as the family doctor or health visitor, should accompany the parent during the interview.

The coroner or other investigative agency

Much depends upon the attitudes and awareness of the medico-legal investigative authority so far as the amount of mental trauma to the parent is concerned. This has greatly improved in Britain and North America over the few decades in which the true nature of cot death has become more common knowledge – again mainly due to the campaigning efforts of the voluntary organisations concerned with the welfare of parents.

In former years, coroners – almost always lawyers without medical training – would hold inquests on victims of SIDS, because the post-mortem examinations then generally recorded a cause of death other than natural disease, such as 'suffocation', 'overlaying' or 'inhalation of vomit'. One such coroner was reported in the press as being proud of having held hundreds of such inquests, which he erroneously felt had furthered the understanding of infant deaths. In actual fact, this practice caused untold extra distress to parents, especially the mothers. There were many coroners who tried to handle matters as sympathetically as they could, but they were hamstrung by the law, which required an inquest (a public enquiry) to be held on all deaths other than those due to certified natural disease.

Other coroners – now thankfully almost, but not quite, defunct – were openly critical of mothers, sometimes to the point of public abuse. The author has had a number of reports of women reduced to tears or near collapse in the witness box of a coroner's court in years gone by, while the coroner chided them about the dangers of soft pillows in the cot or the leaving of a feeding bottle with the infant. Several acute anxiety states can be directly traced to this unjustifiable criticism. One of the most energetic fund-raisers for one of the voluntary organisations was a grandmother who saw her daughter turned into a wreck of self-reproach for almost a year following the castigatory comments of a non-medical coroner at an entirely unnecessary inquest.

In England and Wales, where the coroner system is at its strongest, the position has improved out of all recognition during the past decade or so. Inquests are seldom held, due partly to changes in the law which give coroners far greater discretion in dispensing with inquests, but also because of strenuous efforts by organisations such as the British Guild and the Foundation, who campaigned in the early 1970s for the term 'sudden infant death syndrome' to be accepted by the Registrar-General of Births and Deaths and the Coroners' Society as well as the College of Pathologists as a natural disease process, even if the exact pathological nature was still obscure.

Some of the old public inquests on cot deaths were little short of scandalous, especially when such proceedings were mal-reported in the local press by reporters who understood nothing of the medical background and who frequently wrote distorted accounts of the evidence, usually printed under misleading headlines such as 'Baby Death Remains Mysterious' or 'Mother Quizzed over Mystery Death'.

The press contributed appreciably to the aura of suspicion and uncertainty which hung over SIDS and frequently led to confusion with the then emerging battered baby or child abuse syndrome. Gossip of neighbours was strengthened by local or even national newspaper reports and hurt to parents was deepened. Anxiety, withdrawal and self-recrimination increased in the mother and some families not uncommonly moved house after the tragedy, not only because the dwelling had such sad associations, but sometimes because they felt hostility from neighbours.

The increasing practice of pathologists to certify the death as some natural disease, even when they did not use the words sudden infant death syndrome, allowed coroners to avoid inquests. Terms like 'acute bronchiolitis', 'acute capillary bronchitis' or 'acute tracheo-bronchitis', though scientifically rarely justified, were a let-out for the coroner, who could sign out the case on a Form B without inquest. Later, many pathologists began using the SIDS terminology, either alone or linked with the previous, if tenuous, pathological title and this is the position today.

Although some coroners were as knowledgeable, objective and sympathetic as possible, the very fact of a public inquisition – one of the terms used for an inquest – was to reinforce the distress and feelings of self-reproach in the mother. She was exposed to an unwelcome amount of public scrutiny at a time when she needed to work out her grief in private. Sometimes she was obliged to re-live the harrowing details of the last hours of life and the finding of the dead child – all this within days of the event. From numerous letters received from parents by the supporting organisations, there can be no doubt at all that some coroners' enquiries have been directly responsible for driving some mothers into an acute anxiety state or depressive illness, some of which had suicidal tendencies.

Fortunately, this situation is all but at an end in the English system, but it must serve as a warning to other medico-legal investigative systems which may not yet have had to deal with the problem in countries where improvement in child mortality and greater investigation of deaths will require greater attention to infant deaths in future.

5 · Coping with the death

The reaction of parents to a sudden infant death can be very variable. Some appear to cope extremely well and to go about their usual routine in what appears to be a normal way. Others are completely shattered and some are reduced to a helpless state for many months. In between, there is a whole spectrum of response, though outward appearances are not always an accurate indicator of the emotional turmoil within.

The whole subject of grieving is complex and not fully understood. Attitudes towards death have changed in recent years – indeed it is now sometimes called 'the last taboo', having replaced sexual matters as the area which is glossed over and not spoken about in modern society.

Any study of bereavement following the sudden infant death has to comprise the whole family and not just the mother. There is naturally a tendency to concentrate upon the maternal response, but SIDS affects the whole unit including other children however small, as well as the father. There are also ramifications to more distant members of the family, especially grandparents of the SIDS and brothers and sisters of the parents, especially if any of these are actually resident in the home.

Because of this tendency to make death taboo – especially the death of a child – open reactions may be stifled and thus prolonged. Often the whole system works against the natural release of grief. A dead child is rapidly removed from the house if it is certified dead there. The funeral home is now the usual respository for all our dead, rather than retaining them in the home. Commonly the child is taken to hospital where it is certified dead and frequently taken rapidly from the parents without even the opportunity to say a farewell. The routines of the mortuary and identification are sterile and efficient and everything seems to be done to mechanise and depersonalise the loss. Though sedation of a distracted parent in the initial stages may be humane and necessary, prolonged sedation merely dulls the senses and drags out the period available for the release of grief.

Even some counselling is misdirected, in that there sometimes tends to be an emphasis on forgetting the dead child and making a fresh start as soon as possible with a speedy new pregnancy. The loss of the traditional extended family with numerous relatives on hand to support the bereaved parents has resulted in an isolated nuclear group with little opportunity or inclination to talk out the catastrophe. This is one area in which parent groups can act as a substitute for the extended family, as long as the supportive actions are not drawn out into an unnecessarily long and potentially morbid ritual.

The mother

As Sylvia Limerick, Welfare and Information Chairman of the Foundation, has pointed out in one of her expert articles on counselling, at the peak time for SIDS – about three months – the mother is still recovering from her pregnancy and making post-natal adjustments with attendant hormonal changes. This is a very vulnerable time from the emotional aspect and the mother may well be relatively exhausted with the early weeks of motherhood and night feeds. Her bonding relationship with the baby has had time to grow as it begins to establish its identity as a personality. The baby has survived pregnancy and birth and has escaped gross handicap. The mother, at the same time that she is tired and emotionally fragile, is blossoming into the pride of motherhood and so death is all the more cruel in that it suddenly strikes at the very time of what should be the peak of enjoyment for the mother.

On finding her baby dead, even though some instinct often tells her that her child has gone, a mother may be invaded by a numbing disbelief. This may last long after the doctor has confirmed the fact of death. For a very variable time, perhaps weeks in duration, the mother may think that she hears the baby cry and starts up to go to it. She may physically ache to hold it again and mothers have said that their arms seem to want to hug it of their own volition.

Reactions are enormously variable, including the well-adjusted and practical woman whose apparent self-composure from the very beginning may even lead others to suspect a certain hardness and shallowness of emotion. This is invariably a façade and seems to be more common among self-sufficient, often well-educated women who have or have had a career of their own. A counsellor can sometimes never get behind this mask; indeed, many such self-reliant mothers never present themselves for support. One wonders whether such outward control and suppression of grief may not sometimes be undesirable, spinning the hidden suffering out over a longer period.

At the other extreme are the mothers who literally go to pieces, though thankfully this is usually a short-term phase. A very few pass from this condition into a chronic anxiety state and those who do so may have been helped along the way by some unkind or injudicious comment from an official concerned in the disposal of the death or some unguarded remark by a relative or friend.

A common description is one given by a mother to the effect that she 'felt as if she was losing her mind'. The enormity of the event seems for a time to interfere with logical thought, especially if the hallucinations of hearing the baby's cry or the physical feeling of holding the child strike the mother as being almost supernatural. Her mind may be almost totally occupied with a repetitive replay of the death and all the events associated with it. This period may be worsened by the absence of any available outlet for her true feelings. The mother may feel totally alone and even abandoned, unable in some cases to talk frankly even with her husband. Thoughts of guilt and remorse which chase themselves in an endless circle through her mind are so common as to be almost standard components of the grief, even if the woman does not recognise this herself. When an outlet is at last found – though sometimes it never is – the extent of this pent-up emotion can then be truly appreciated. When she discovers a counsellor, a member of a befriending organisation, an understanding doctor or health visitor or a really sympathetic friend or relative, the dam of her mind bursts and all the stifled thoughts and terrors can come pouring out.

In the innumerable letters written to the various voluntary organisations, this outpouring, amounting almost to fantasy in some cases, is so very obvious. The author has had up to 18 letters in a single day in the bad old days when so many mothers were totally ignorant of any facts at all about SIDS. A mother may write a 20-page letter giving a point-by-point account of every feed for days before the death and a minute description of every cough and sniffle that the child made. Similar release is made in face-to-face talks to counsellors or friends, lowering the dangerous flood-level of torturing thoughts. Many mothers have said later that it was this point of release, either in talking or even writing to a sympathetic listener, that marked the start of the road to recovery.

More especially in the days before the early 1970s, when SIDS was almost an unknown quantity, even to many doctors, mothers found that the worst burden to bear was finding that no one understood. The difficulty then was to find someone who knew anything about sudden infant death syndrome or who had even heard of it! Even if the actual event of SIDS was dimly appreciated, even fewer knew anything about the mental turmoil which the mother was suffering. Bereaved mothers, when they eventually found one of the few counsellors who existed in those days, were pathetically grateful when they could unburden themselves to someone who had some knowledge of the syndrome and of the trauma it inflicted on families.

Even those without any medical knowledge were a boon in just providing a sympathetic ear because the major need then was to obtain some mental catharsis by pouring out the story and the hidden fears. Finding another parent who had suffered the same tragedy was very useful, as it is today, as parents could share the feelings which were quite incomprehensible to those who had not gone through the same trauma. This was the origin of the Guilds in the United States before doctors came to play any significant role in the process.

Within the proviso that parent group therapy should not be so prolonged or so emotionally intense as to become a self-perpetuating ritual, the influence of what might be called a 'peer group' may be very useful indeed. Commonly the mother does not need all that much counselling in the practical sense of explanations and advice for the future, but merely needs an ear into which to release her frustrations and anxieties, especially about the possibilities of her own actions or neglect having contributed to the death.

It was the isolation that was so unbearable, according to the more articulate SIDS parents who later discussed their acute stage of bereavement with their counsellor. 'No one knew what I was going through' was the common cry from the heart. 'They told me to pull myself together' was another, and 'They thought that I had killed my baby' was a not infrequent complaint from those who could find no one who knew anything about sudden infant death and seemed surrounded by those who were frankly suspicious, sometimes prompted by misleading newspapers reports of inquests. Quite often, normally sympathetic neighbours and relatives would confuse SIDS with the battered child syndrome, which in the 1960s was also bursting upon the public's attention. The author well recalls a mother telling him that when she found her baby dead her first panic-stricken reaction was to telephone her mother whose immediate response was to cry down the phone, 'My God, what have you done to him?'

The father

The inhibitions about death are so deeply rooted in modern society that even the husband is often less of a support than might be imagined. Of course there are numerous exceptions to this statement and many fathers are a tower of strength to their wives, even though they themselves may be grieved to distraction.

Some fathers have told those offering support that they themselves did not want to bring up the subject because it might distress their wives even more – saying this usually when rejecting any counselling for the pair of them. The husband is traditionally the strong, silent member of the partnership, though those working with support organisations or as individual counsellors often see the opposite face of the coin. Social conventions tend to deprive the father of the opportunity to display his grief that is traditionally afforded to women.

Much less attention has been paid to the father in SIDS tragedies, yet many opportunities have occurred to discover that paternal grief may be profound, though better suppressed – if 'better' is an appropriate word in these circumstances. It is true that the father is in a less vulnerable position than his wife, not having been so immersed in the everyday routine of feeding, bathing, dressing and caring for the child that so totally wraps up the woman's way of life. However active a part a father may take in bringing up their child, the bonds that connect mother and child can never be as strong for the man. In most cases, he is the breadwinner at this time of their life and is out of the house for much of the most active hours of parental care. He is also more likely to have outside distractions with his work, mixing with and meeting people outside the home far more than the mother, who may be semi-imprisoned at home during this stage of the baby's development.

All these facts combine to make it unlikely that he will experience the unnerving after death experiences of hearing the child's cry and of aching to hold it to the breast, which can so upset the mother. This said, there is still no doubt that the father has been relatively displaced in the post-death situation and counsellors should always talk to him to see what state of affairs exists with respect to his feelings, hopes and fears.

Sometimes a cot death will cause a serious rift in the marriage. The husband, especially if ill-informed and deprived of advice, may openly or covertly blame the mother for the loss of *his* child. The rift may be temporary and may be healed by good counselling, but not infrequently it remains and may even lead to a complete breakdown of the relationship, though where this happens there is usually some other evidence of a failing bond, the SIDS being the last straw or catalyst that widens the rift. The author has knowledge of several families where the death of the infant seemed to be the start of a breach leading to actual divorce. It is essential, especially where the mother is convinced of her own guilt in some imagined neglect that led to the death, that not only she, but her husband, be firmly reassured of the natural causes of cot death. Once the seed of doubt is planted and germinates unchecked in the husband's mind, later counselling may not be effective.

In some instances the father reacts in a most negative way immediately after a sudden infant death by denying the mother access to support and counselling. A few cases have been seen in which even tentative offers of help and advice have been brusquely rejected – sometimes aggressively – by the father, who acts a supposedly protective role in keeping any reminder of the tragedy from his wife. Little can be done by counsellors in this unfortunate situation, though fortunately it is uncommon.

Brothers and sisters

The other children in the family – the siblings – may be profoundly affected by the sudden death of their infant companion. A variety of reactions may be seen, from indifference to outright fear of suffering the same fate. Others are plagued by guilty feelings that their thoughts of dislike or jealousy or even some trivial acts of teasing or disturbing the baby on some recent occasion may have caused the death. Some siblings begin to have nightmares or start bed-wetting after the infant's death. Others become pathologically clinging and dependent, an index of their fear of the death coming back to claim them. Yet other children seem to become unusually naughty or have temper tantrums, generally a sign of their seeking added attention.

The brothers and sisters need careful handling if symptoms appear and the help of the doctor, health visitor or in extreme cases, a child psychiatrist may be needed. Explanations by the parents should be as accurate and explicit as age and understanding allows. Fanciful explanations as to the fate of the baby, made with motives of sparing their feelings, may be counter-productive. It has been reported that saying 'The baby has been taken by Jesus' has led the sibling to think of Jesus as 'some rapacious baby-snatcher'. The same writers, with massive experience in Sheffield, relate that another child, on being told that baby 'had gone to live in God's house', took to visiting churches in the hope of finding his sister.

It seems preferable to explain that the baby died of a rare disease, which affects very few babies of a very young age and that it will not happen to older children. This can only be done with brothers or sisters old enough to follow the explanation, who will in any case be out of the SIDS risk age. It is said that a surviving twin needs special counselling as though they are so young the loss can be appreciated even at six months, and may lead to insecurity as the survivor gets older.

Grandparents

The grandparents may be severely shocked by a cot death. A grandchild may be very precious, especially as it often forms a replay of their own parenthood, a kind of rejuvenation where they are enjoying their own younger years through their second generation child. To lose this child suddenly and unexpectedly can upset them greatly and there is the added sorrow of seeing the desolation of their own child and spouse, the infant's parents.

Grandparents may, in fact, become most ardent campaigners in the fight against SIDS and not infrequently become active members of a voluntary organisation devoted to cot death research. The Foundation for the Study of Infant Deaths was largely founded through the determination of such a bereaved grandparent who financed a medical conference on cot death in Cambridge in 1970, which led directly to the forming of the FSID.

They may, however, contribute to some of the troubles which develop after a sudden infant death by being over-critical, either overtly or by insinuation, of the care the mother gave to the child and the standard of mothering. This naturally is more common on the part of the paternal grandparents. This can sow seeds of family discord and cases are known in which the grandparents have retreated entirely from contact with the family after a row with the mother and/or father. Though grandparents can be very supportive, the grandmother may feel that her superior (if outdated) knowledge of mothercraft entitles her to lecture her daughter-in-law on what she should have done or should not have done to avoid the tragedy. This is a recipe for disaster as far as family friction is concerned.

Support for the parents

Once the initial shock has passed, there is overwhelming grief and a sense of bewilderment. It is at this stage that support is needed and many parents have said later that they felt that such support was lacking in the very early stages after the tragedy. Some support agencies have deliberately held off until several days have passed or perhaps even a fortnight or more, thinking that their help will be more acceptable once the acute shock of the death has passed off. This may be so in some cases, but it seems the more general opinion of parents, who have suffered the loss of a child, is that early intervention should be offered.

Support can come from a number of directions:

1. *Health visitors* or equivalent professional health care personnel have a primary role in reaching the parents during the acute stages of their bereavement. In Britain the health visitor service is a highly skilled occupation provided by dedicated women who are originally trained as nurses, but who later qualify as professional counsellors in the home environment. In some areas in Britain there are special

paediatric health visitors and, where a particular interest is taken in the SIDS problem, there may be one or more health visitors with special responsibility for this type of counselling. In the Sheffield pilot study there were several health visitors whose sole task was to visit the bereaved relatives. Their role is a primary one to explain and comfort, but they also act as liaison between other types of health care which may be required.

2. *The family physician* is a vital link in the counselling chain, but one which is all too frequently lacking or deficient. Where there is a general practitioner who is both knowledgeable and conscientious about SIDS counselling, his help can be invaluable. Not only has he a prior relationship with the family which gives him a unique link, but he is in a better position to explain the medical aspects of sudden infant death with an authoritative voice. He also has extensive powers and connections with other health care facilities which can help the family to cope with the multiple problems that may arise from their tragedy. Parents have said that a visit from their doctor immediately after the tragedy can be a most supportive event. Some general practitioners return several times on the day of the tragedy to see what can be done and make regular and frequent visits thereafter. Unfortunately, it is all too often the experience of parents that the general practitioner comes reluctantly or not at all.

3. *A paediatrician* will not normally enter the situation unless there is some specific arrangement made. Because of the lack of available counselling and the frequent inability or unwillingness of the family physician to assist significantly in counselling, arrangements have been made, mainly via the voluntary associations described below, to have certain consultant paediatricians in each area in Britain available for consultation, if the parents so wish. The British Paediatric Association invited from among its members those who were interested and willing to agree to see parents and explain and counsel on the many problems associated with SIDS. In the

earlier years of the more recent interest in SIDS, paediatricians themselves were not all that familiar with the syndrome because it rarely occurs in hospital and, unless paediatricians developed a particular interest from studying the world literature, they may not have been particularly expert in the topic. They naturally had considerable expertise in the general field of counselling in paediatric matters and their advice was most valuable; it seems doubtful if this facility has been used very much, except in those cases where other forms of counselling appear to have had little effect – mainly in the acute anxiety states and depressions which have gone on for a longer time after the tragedy than is usual.

4. *The pathologist* is also a source of counselling but, in general, many pathologists are reluctant to become involved with the parents. Probably partly because of inclination, many pathologists have chosen the scientific and laboratory aspects of their careers because they were not greatly attracted to clinical work with its inevitable doctor-patient dialogue. Though it is of considerable advantage for the pathologist who conducted the post-mortem examination to be able to talk to the parents about the results and implications, many pathologists are reluctant or even adamantly opposed to any interview with parents. An editorial by Dr Lester Adelson of Cleveland, Ohio, drew attention to this fact and strongly advocated that the pathologist should be available to the parents. The editorial was entitled 'Physician to the bereaved' and concerned other types of death as well as SIDS cases, though this was his main concern. Following this leader, the present author wrote a similar recommendation in the *British Medical Journal*, exhorting his colleagues to be more ready to speak to relatives when they so wish. Though it can be a delicate matter for the doctor who has carried out an extensive examination on the body of a cherished child, to discuss the matter dispassionately with the parents, a careful and sensitive approach can avoid any awkwardness. The parents almost invariably seem to derive considerable benefit from an authoritative explana-

tion, based on facts gained from the most fundamental of evidence. The pathologist is also often most aware of recent developments in the research field in SIDS and this has helped in putting across the most up-to-date explanation of what has happened.

The role of the voluntary organisations concerned with sudden infant death is a matter of extreme importance. Something of their history must be considered to appreciate how they came into being.

VOLUNTARY ORGANISATIONS

In the United States of America some 20 years ago a number of bereaved parents became so exasperated by the complete lack of information or appreciation of their plight that they banded together into several isolated groups, generally called guilds. These were formed gradually in a number of cities and States across the country, being totally self-help organisations at the outset. Parents who had suffered the tragedy of crib death met together to exchange experiences – mostly harrowing – and began to look for newly bereaved parents to help. Knowing the total isolation, bewilderment and lack of information or constructive sympathy available, these parents went out to look for those who were suffering the same trouble, to give them something of what they themselves had lacked.

In the early stages very few doctors or health care people were involved but gradually the guilds drew in physicians, paediatricians and pathologists so that medical expertise began to be stimulated.

It is probably due almost entirely to the efforts of these guilds that the present upsurge in research and epidemiology has taken place. Whereas before the 1950s there was virtually nothing in medical literature about SIDS, there is now a massive reference collection well in excess of 2000 titles. This snowball effect can be traced back to the activity of these dedicated parents in the United States, whose activities spread both across their own nation and into Canada and across to Britain and Northern Europe.

The American guilds eventually polarised into several groups, the largest being the National Foundation for Sudden Infant Death (NFSID). These groups, both large and small, produced useful leaflets which were very explanatory in themselves and were also an introduction for newly-bereaved parents to the actual guilds. In addition to their counselling activities, the guilds began to raise money for research and, just as importantly, began social and political pressure for allocation of public funds for research.

The medical spin-off of this activity began to accumulate and eventually a series of international conferences was held, the first being in Seattle in September 1963. This was followed by another meeting in Seattle in 1969. In 1970 there was a further symposium in Cambridge, England, and in 1974 the Canadian Foundation held another meeting in Toronto. Though these were the high spots of international co-operation, there have been many other smaller meetings and extensive work done in the interim. In the United States the National Institute of Health, through its National Institute of Child Health and Human Development, have taken a great interest in SIDS and have produced a series of publications on research and planning.

The American experience of parents' guilds moved across the Atlantic in the late 1960s and early 1970s. Two quite separate organisations began in Britain almost simultaneously – the British Guild for Sudden Infant Death Study, started by the author of this book and his wife in 1970, and the Foundation for the Study of Infant Deaths, started in London. This latter organisation has now become the most active in the world and, as there was no point in duplicating information services and leaflets in a country the size of Britain, the British Guild merged with it.

The Foundation came about virtually by a single tragedy. The grandmother of an infant victim wished to donate some money towards research into SIDS and the late Dr Francis Camps, the well-known London forensic pathologist, suggested that the best means of using this donation was to hold a seminar in Cambridge on sudden infant death. From this the Foundation was established with Sir Max Aitken as President. The Foundation has revolutionised both the counselling and research aspects of SIDS in Britain and, indeed, in many other countries because its enthusiasm and expertise have spread in many directions. Almost all research at the moment is either funded, or supported in other ways, by the Foundation and a small permanently staffed office in London is available to provide information and counselling. In addition, the Foundation has numerous associated parent groups around Britain to which newly bereaved parents can be directed if they wish to talk with other individual parents who not only understand but can help them express their feelings as well as being able to give practical advice based on their own experience. Such friendships can extend to giving support with subsequent children.

It also provides reference material for the medical profession and issues guidelines for infant care and the handling of SIDS tragedies in hospital accident departments, to name but a small part of their activities.

These then are the facilities available to parents – if they are aware of them. This was one of the earliest problems when the Foundation and other organisations were established. Parents knew nothing of any organised assistance – and indeed knew nothing of the existence of SIDS until it struck them personally. The problem was to make the availability of such advice and counselling known to the general population. Things got off to a slow start and it was mainly by word of mouth and by newspaper journalism that the message slowly spread. Some magazines were strangely reluctant to publish anything about SIDS. A well-known women's magazine rejected the offer of an article on the grounds that it would 'frighten the mothers'. Some years later, when the whole problem of SIDS became general knowledge, the same magazine accepted a similar article, falling in line with many other more progressive publications.

When the organisations managed to get some newspaper publicity in those earlier years, each new item of news brought in a fresh surge of letters. Parents, who had either recently or earlier suffered SIDS in their family, suddenly became aware that they had not been alone after all – that there were some people who actually knew of this terrible scourge and were willing to talk about it. The response was amazing and on some days after the publication of a national newspaper article, the postbag for even a small organisation like the British Guild was overwhelming.

As years went by and publicity about SIDS became more commonplace there was a noticeable change in the requests for information. Initially it was totally a parent-oriented matter, but medical and health care personnel became much more curious and receptive. Innumerable requests came from doctors, health visitors, family clinics, midwives, nurse training schools and nurses themselves for information about sudden infant death. Guild and Foundation literature went out in larger amounts not only to individual parents, but to clinics, hospitals, health centres and later to coroners' officers. This last group became very important, because coroners' officers dealt with virtually every cot death parent in the country. They were therefore in a central and primary position to offer the first contact to parents if they wished to take it up. Nowadays most coroners' officers have supplies of the Foundation leaflet available to give to bereaved parents very shortly after the tragedy. The mother or father can then decide whether they wish to pursue matters, either for further written information, telephone conversation with someone knowledgeable or contact with a parent group.

Contact with such an organisation is, of course, entirely voluntary: never would a counsellor force attention upon a parent. Not infrequently it happens that a mother – and perhaps more often a father – actively resists the attempt at counselling or even advice. This appears to be due to some deep-seated attempt at self-protection, on the principle that if the whole episode is shut out and denied it can be imagined never to have existed. On rare occasions, a father has contacted the counselling organisation in a most forthright and sometimes aggressive way, objecting to the supply of leaflets and warning off any further attempts at contact – which naturally is immediately complied with.

Most parents, however, are only too anxious to get further information and often to unburden themselves to someone who is sympathetically inclined. So often, it is not counselling or even much information that is required, but merely the opportunity to have a shoulder to cry on, which appears to have a cathartic effect. This can be done either by letter or direct contact, and much of the mailbags of the organisations consists of such letters, describing the circumstances in great detail. Many of these letters express utter relief merely at the fact that someone else exists who appreciates the feelings of emptiness and loss, to say nothing of bewilderment, which the parents suffer. This knowledge of appreciation of their plight in itself is frequently seen to have a very beneficial effect.

Many such parents never contact the counselling organisation again. It would appear that this first unburdening is sufficient to allow them to return gradually to a normal state of mind after the usual grieving period has elapsed. The spectrum includes parents from those who apparently showed little emotion and no disruption of their life's routine to those who were frantically distressed to the point of suicide or who went into an anxiety state, which lasted for many months on some occasions.

Even such severe cases seem to recover spontaneously within a year, apart of course from the tiny minority who develop some serious psychological disturbance. The vast majority slowly return to normal, this process being greatly accelerated if a new pregnancy occurs. Counselling and contact with parent groups is a potent source of acceleration for this return to normal and it is noticeable that even severely upset parents tend to vanish from the sight of the counselling organisation within a matter of months. Often the newly-bereaved parents channel their grief into frantically enthusiastic work for the organisation, or in developing local parent groups, or in fund-raising activities. It is noticeable that these activists very often seem to work out their need to participate and, within months or a year, quietly subside into inactivity and slide back into their normal pattern of life.

The type of primary information offered to newly bereaved parents can be seen from some examples from several of the organisations on both sides of the Atlantic. They naturally tend to be repetitive as the facts on which they are based are identical and there is naturally much cross-fertilisation between one organisation and another. In addition, the Foundation for the Study of Infant Deaths offer more extensive advice in relation to future children and the general care of babies, anticipating that after a family loses one child by SIDS it will naturally be markedly over-protective of the next infant, the fear of a further SIDS always hovering near.

One of the inevitable questions asked of counsellors by SIDS parents is 'Will it happen to my next baby – is it hereditary?' Thankfully it can be said that there is no hereditary basis for cot death that has so far been detected. Counsellors can tell relatives that the risk of a cot death occurring in future infants is very small. Recent studies have shown that the risk is about three times that of an unaffected family, this figure should be tempered by reversing the arithmetic and explaining that of every 500 babies subsequently born to previous SIDS parents, 497 will survive.

Though, until quite recently, it was customary to deny any increased risk whatsoever, it is now perhaps better to slightly modify this assurance but simultaneously link it with the previous statement about the very small number of post-SIDS recurrences. Multiple cot deaths have been reported and, where two occur in a family, then it is usually ascribable to this mathematical risk. However, some sensational press reports have given accounts of three, four and even five cot deaths in a family. These are almost without exception not true SIDS, but must be some familial or hereditary inborn disease which has not been recognised, at least by the newspaper. In counselling, therefore, it is legitimate in the circumstances to reassure the parents that the risk of a subsequent tragedy of the same nature is little greater than if the first one had not occurred.

Counselling

Of the two practical things that can be done in the whole sad affair of sudden infant death, one is prevention (see Chapter 6) and the other is counselling of relatives after a tragedy has taken place. Counselling is one of our greatest growth industries and during the sociological revolution that has occurred since the last war, many official, semi-official and voluntary organisations have mushroomed to provide counselling for almost every conceivable personal problem that can be imagined.

Counselling is a convenient though perhaps rather grand word for constructive, objective, sympathetic advice. In the context of cot death, counselling has been carried on at least since the time of Solomon, whose advice in the dispute between the two mothers as to which infant had survived the sudden death, was to order the survivor to be cut in half, rapidly revealing the true mother! Less drastic, but much more practical, advice has come from all sorts of people ever since. Undoubtedly, for thousands of years the bulk of advice and support came from other members of the extended family around the mother. No doubt much of it was wrong, critical and even malicious, but in ages where infant mortality was massive, perhaps guilt was correspondingly less. These days, with small families, often very independent and isolated, and with the pressures far greater with each infant death because of the modern low level of mortality, the need for support has become much greater.

A lot of it still comes from relatives, perhaps far more than we think, for those who come to the attention of both the professional and the voluntary counsellors are often those who lack enough family support. But, for a variety of reasons already discussed, the prime needs for a large proportion of SIDS parents are sympathy, understanding, explanation and advice.

These are needed *urgently* in many cases and *soon* in almost all, whatever the source. One of the lessons learned almost incidentally in some of the research surveys into SIDS was that parents want *immediate* help, not a visit in a fortnight or a month. There was a tendency some years ago to delay any counselling approach for a week or two, often until after the funeral was over. For the best of motives it was felt that the family, especially the mother, would be more receptive to help once the initial acute grief was over. But responses from parents, in letters, in discussions and in surveys such as that held by the Foundation, showed quite clearly that most parents wanted sympathy and advice straight after the tragedy. Many, in fact, were sufficiently balanced again in a fortnight not to be in much need of support, though they were still anxious for hard facts in the form of explanations about the nature of the condition and the specific findings in their own baby's case.

We have already mentioned the various sources of counselling which are or should be available. These include the family's own general physician who, if he is assiduous, can be about the most effective of all in giving comfort and authoritative advice. Probably the health visitor, in the British context, has the greatest role to play because this really is her job, without the numerous diversions that afflict the general practitioner.

The health visitor, especially one involved specifically in paediatric work – or even a special SIDS officer, as is available in a few places – has the training, motivation and access to have a very effective role. She may well have been visiting the family previously and have an existing rapport with them, which can be a great asset when having to continue in a counselling role over a cot death. There is a danger here, which has surfaced occasionally, due to lack of communication. It has happened that the health visitor has arrived at a house on a routine visit, unaware that a SIDS tragedy has struck since her last attendance. This can be a situation fraught with embarrassment and tension and it is therefore essential for every area to have a foolproof system of notification between all members of a health care team. The same system of communication should make health visitors aware within hours that a SIDS has taken place so that she can make the initial visit as soon as possible, certainly not later than the following day. In Cardiff (South Glamorgan), all perinatal deaths are monitored by a working party consisting of paediatricians, community physicians, health visitors, pathologists, nurses, etc. They have established an early warning system, based on the coroner's officer, pathologist and hospital accident department, which alerts those needing to know as soon as a SIDS occurs. As a result the health visitor is able to get to the family very early – exactly what SIDS parents say they need.

Several visits are needed; it is found that during the early meetings the parents, though very glad of the support, do not take in explanations. At later visits, they ask the same questions again and have more chance of retaining the answers once the acute phase is over.

The health visitor, perhaps even better than the doctor, can discuss matters such as the formalities of the coroner's investigation, registration of death, the funeral and other practicalities, which sometimes seem to be the only things to surface in the numbed minds of the parents, before the longer-term problems of grief, longing, self-recrimination, etc., take full hold on their emotions. The ministrations of the health visitor may be needed over a long time – many months, in fact. Quite a significant number of SIDS parents move house to get away from the unhappy associations, or neighbours, and it is important that the health visitor does not lose track of them. If they go to a distant area, she should make arrangements to hand them on to a health visitor in that district.

Sometimes a community physician, usually one involved in child health, may also take part in counselling, either at the home or sometimes by appointment at his office. Less often, a community nurse or even the midwife who delivered the child may have a useful role in counselling – it usually depends on who has the best rapport with the mother and on the harder facts of availability.

We have talked about the very important role in counselling of the charitable and voluntary organisations such as the various guilds and the Foundation for the Study of Infant Deaths. Their first contacts are usually through leaflets or by word of mouth from some relative, nurse or doctor. In some areas, guild members actively look for newly bereaved parents, either in newspaper reports or death notices or by some contact in the health care team.

This more active approach needs to be used with caution because some families may rebuff any such approaches and a few may be distressed or even resentful of what they feel is an intrusion on their privacy at a time of intense grief. On the whole, it seems better to seed the ground with helpful literature, giving addresses and telephone numbers where further help may readily be obtained. The more official counselling will (or should) be made available to parents via the health care team so a more passive approach is justified. This applies to the areas and countries where the system is well organised; perhaps a more aggressive approach is justified elsewhere – at least, in making sure that the initial literature is made available.

THE CONTENT OF COUNSELLING

This is a very personal matter and no detailed rules can be laid down. By selection, temperament and training, professional counsellors like health visitors, paediatricians and, to a lesser extent, general physicians, have a sensitivity, a kind of mental radar which detects what the parents need and what they are trying to extract from their advisor.

Every SIDS situation is different in that, apart from the fairly universal need to know about 'What is it?', 'What causes it?', 'What did I do wrong?', 'Was it my fault?', 'Will it happen again?', there are more personal matters which vary from case to case. Common ones, perhaps at a later stage in counselling, include problems about re-housing, the absence of the risk of SIDS to other children in the family, death grants and funeral expenses, about a new baby, marriage or family troubles, changing doctor, and host of matters from feeding the other children to getting a new job.

Many of these matters stray from the SIDS problem into the field of general social work, but most arise directly or otherwise from the disruption caused by the tragedy. If the counsellor begins to feel that they are getting beyond her capabilities then at least she can direct the parent to another more specialised source of help.

The bulk of the queries, especially in the first few weeks, tend to be repetitive and along the lines already discussed at length. Often there are no real questions, just the need to have a sympathetic listener, someone to whom the mother can pour out her pent-up memories, worries and fears. Answers to questions often fail to sink in and the counsellor must have great patience to avoid frustration at having to repeat apparently simple facts which have failed to make any impact upon the confused mind of the parent.

6 · Can SIDS be prevented?

There are two main lines possible in the attack on the tragic problem of sudden infant death: the mechanism by which individual deaths occur can be interrupted, or a general attack can be made upon the predisposing factors.

The first depends upon correct identification of the defect in the body systems which lead to the death. Unless we have successfully worked out exactly what goes wrong in each infant victim, then a specific regime of prevention is unlikely to be successful. At the present time, the majority of researchers feel that the sleep apnoea-hypoxia is most likely to be either the whole truth or a substantial part of the truth, though there are those who quite legitimately say that the causes lie elsewhere. Therefore, at present, strenuous efforts are being made to devise methods of breaking the vicious circle of respiratory depression and the associated abnormalities.

The second approach is what one might call epidemiological, that is, study of a very large number of SIDS to discover what kinds of baby are prone to fall victim to the condition. This also has been done and it must be said that there are some difficulties in marrying the two approaches, in that it is hard to see how some of the factors thrown up by epidemiological surveys could possibly be related to the apnoea-hypoxia supposition. This only goes to confirm that SIDS is an extraordinarily complex problem and that we are deluding ourselves if we think there is a simple explanation and an equally simple method of prevention. Someone reading this book in 10 years time might be amazed at how blind and ignorant we were, just as we tend to patronise those who thought that malaria was due to the fumes emitted from marshes.

Nevertheless, we have to deal with the situation as it stands in our time and, taking the two approaches just mentioned, the possible ways of defeating this scourge are set out below.

Sleep apnoea-hypoxia

This was discussed fully in Chapter 3 but, to recapitulate, the theory is that SIDS occurs because a baby with a tendency towards abnormally long periods of cessation of breathing during sleep, becomes short of oxygen. Because of various other factors, including the possibility of nasal narrowing, difficulty in mouth breathing, constriction of the back of the throat and perhaps some narrowing at vocal cord level, this shortage of oxygen increases. This in turn perpetuates the apnoea and causes slowing of the heart with eventual stoppage, so that the child actually dies of cardiorespiratory failure.

Obviously, anything that will prevent this descending spiral will prevent the baby's death. It is probable that if all babies were watched all the time, any long period of apnoea could be frustrated by stimulating the child by simple means such as handling or prodding or anything which would break the vicious circle. As mentioned earlier, it is obviously quite impracticable to watch all babies all the time, especially as we are seeking only one baby out of every 500. Therefore methods must be devised to refine this observation process.

The first and obvious thing to do is to devise some mechanical device which will automatically warn of the cessation of breathing for more than a predetermined time. In other words, we need an apnoea alarm. This is a relatively straightforward piece of electrical engineering, though to make it foolproof is a different matter. The older types consisted of an inflated cuff around the infant's chest, but several more sophisticated models are now available. One consists of a special mattress containing a sensitive electronic device, the Lewin mattress. Another can be taped to the infant's skin and a new one measures the change in curvature of the abdominal wall, which moves as the diaphragm goes up and down. These alarms can be pre-set to give a warning (by bell or light) when breathing movements of the chest and abdominal wall have ceased for a certain length of time, say 20 seconds. There are usually fail-safe mechanisms built into the apparatus – for example, the alarm will sound if the device falls away from the baby.

They may all be liable to faults, which constitute the most serious criticisms of their use. First, they may give false-negative results, in other words, fail to give the alarm when breathing stops for a long time. This may be due to technical faults, but may also occur because the device picks up the heart beat in error for breathing, even though breathing may have stopped. More often, there are false-positive alarms, and these can be very common, but naturally a potent source of terror for parents who hear the alarm go off. This may again be due to wrong adjustment or technical faults, but if the breathing is very shallow, though adequate, the alarm may trigger.

More reliable devices are being produced all the time and the safety factor is increasing. For example, one of the most convenient and safest at the time of writing is the Graseby Dynamics Respiration Monitor MR 10, which consists of a small plastic box with two red warning lights and a loud bleeper. Powered by a small in-built battery, with no mains current or electrical connections to endanger the child, it can be tucked into a corner of the cot. A thin plastic tube connects it to the sensor, which is a little capsule fixed to the baby's stomach wall with adhesive tape. This sensor has a diaphragm which picks up pressure changes occurring as the abdomen moves during breathing and transmits them to the control box through the hollow tube. If the movements stop for more than a pre-determined time, the alarms are triggered. If the sensor falls off the baby, the alarm goes off.

The objection that such an alarm will continue to give a safe signal because the stomach is still moving, even if the upper airway is blocked, has given impetus to research to find ways of detecting actual airflow; such an instrument can be fitted near the nose and will only trigger the alarm if the passage of air through the nostrils ceases; so far, these are rather impractical for small babies, but have been used on older children and adults with breathing problems.

Many parents who have suffered a previous cot death in the family, seem to derive considerable comfort and peace of mind from the use of an apnoea alarm. The MR 10 gives a gentle 'click' at every breath and some mothers have said that this reassuring sound is most welcome. One mother said that she actually managed to finish her housework more quickly when the baby was connected to the alarm, as she merely listened to the clicks as she worked, rather than spending time running anxiously in and out of the room to check if her baby was breathing normally.

The debate continues, sometimes escalating into medical controversy. On balance, it seems that if parents are selected, properly instructed, and supported by emergency back-up facilities, the use of monitors can be a great relief to families who are otherwise likely to suffer chronic apprehension following a previous SIDS tragedy.

There is no doubt that apnoea alarms, which are being improved all the time, do a good job in detecting apnoea. But the question remains, how confident can we be that this is related to SIDS and can it be a significant protection for high-risk babies?

For this is the next point, even assuming that the alarms are reliable indicators – to which babies should they be fitted? Even though one bio-engineer seriously suggested fitting them to all babies in Britain under the age of six months – an economic and ethical non-starter – it has to be accepted that for practical reasons only a very small proportion of infants can be – or need to be – fitted with alarms. These are infants at highest risk because (a) they are known to have had apnoeic and cyanotic attacks –perhaps true near-miss babies; (b) premature and/or under-birth-weight infants who have respiratory troubles, apnoeic or otherwise; or (c) subsequent children born to a family who have already suffered a sudden infant death.

Though these groups are by no means all at risk because of a tendency to apnoea, using these groupings certainly reduces the large low-risk mass to manageable proportions, though again this residual group needs careful study and consideration before apnoea alarms are handed out on a haphazard basis.

When an alarm is decided upon, then a strict back-up regime is necessary to avoid as much harm as good being done. First, where an alarm is used at home the parents must be trained in resuscitatory techniques – it is patently futile to provide the means to detect potentially fatal apnoea if no provision is made for emergency treatment like mouth-to-mouth respiration or the use of a breathing mask and bag. Second, the parents must be fully conversant with the function and usage of the monitor and there must be a cast-iron system of repair and maintenance for the device on a night-and-day basis. Last, the health care team of general practitioner, health visitor, etc., must be fully in the picture and briefed so that they act constructively in any emergency.

Without all these safeguards, the indiscriminate dispensing of alarms – sometimes obtained privately by the parents themselves – is likely to lead to unsatisfactory and possible tragic results.

Even when the provisions are perfect, many experienced doctors are unconvinced that apnoea alarms have any relevance in SIDS and say that if they have any use it is to give some peace of mind to the parents of high-risk infants or to those parents who have previously suffered a cot death in the family.

Controversy exists over the whole question of apnoea monitors, though perhaps not so much between those who believe strongly in their preventive worth and those who think they are useless, but between the convinced and the doubters, who are by no means convinced that there is a protective role. It has been pointed out that perhaps four out of every five SIDS have nothing in their history to suggest that they ever suffered from prolonged sleep apnoea. Others point to the fact that where apnoea is due to obstruction of the air passages – a more dangerous state than cessation of the respiratory drive which moves the chest – the apnoea monitor may not ring. Although the chest may be moving, there will be no tidal air moving in and out of the lungs, so a potentially fatal hypoxia and heart slowing could be well advanced before the alarm went off.

In an effort to clarify the worth or otherwise of alarms, a number of studies are going on at present. One of the largest is that by the major figure in sleep apnoea in relation to SIDS, Dr Alfred Steinschneider in the United States. He is making an extensive survey of thousands of babies in a large study in New York State, which will take several years to complete.

In Britain, the Foundation is naturally very concerned with the problem and held a conference on the subject in Sheffield in 1979, from which investigations flowed and are still going on. At that conference, which attracted many researchers in the field including Dr Steinschneider, all the problems and objections related above were discussed at length. It was shown that some children could stop breathing for as much as 40 seconds and appear none the worse for it. Because obstructive apnoea may cause profound hypoxia (oxygen lack) even though an alarm is not registering any stoppage of chest movement, it was suggested that a cardiac monitor to detect slow heart rate (the first sign of imminent heart failure) might be a more effective monitoring system.

At present there is such a great range of variable breathing patterns in babies both asleep and awake that there is a need to collect a lot of data on normal patterns in babies; this is being done in Britain and elsewhere. Some doctors think it too early to pin our faith on apnoea monitors until we know far more about respiratory physiology; others take a more empirical view and feel that, while we are waiting for this data, efforts should be made to save a few lives.

To try to add more information to the current knowledge, the Foundation for the Study of Infant Deaths is currently organising a practical trial among volunteers from families who have had a SIDS previously. As there is some evidence to suggest that brothers and sisters of SIDS may have a greater tendency to irregular breathing patterns during sleep (though this by no means indicates that they are that much more likely to have the tragedy afflict them), 50 SIDS siblings are being sought for apnoea monitoring at home – naturally with all the back-up prerequisites mentioned earlier. As well as providing valuable information on the frequency of apnoeic episodes, it will also form a parallel trial for another suggested method of preventing potential SIDS in a further 50 brothers or sisters of previous SIDS. This other 50 will not be placed on apnoea alarms, but will be put on a very careful weighing regime as it has been suggested that the pre-SIDS illness period, which so often goes unnoticed, may be detected by a fairly abrupt arrest in the normal weight gain. This approach arose mainly from work in Sheffield, where Professor Emery and his colleagues are convinced that most SIDS had symptoms and signs of illness in the days or weeks before the tragedy. Weight loss may be an indicator that can be relatively easily detected at home; if found, then energetic general medical surveillance and treatment may restore matters to normal. Both these methods are partly directed towards giving parents peace of mind; they will only be applied to families naturally anxious after the loss of a previous child.

The whole question of apnoea alarms is thus wide open at the moment. After the Sheffield conference in 1979 the Foundation issued a statement on their position in the matter, which has not substantially changed at the present time. One paragraph sums up the situation:

> The value of apnoea alarms to prevent sudden unexpected infant deaths is not yet established. The extent, if any, to which prolonged apnoeic spells are the underlying cause of death in otherwise healthy babies is not yet known. Only a small proportion of babies who have died unexpectedly have had a proven history of apnoeic spells. There is therefore insufficient evidence to recommend the widespread use of apnoea alarms for normal babies to prevent cot deaths.

The epidemiological approach

For most of the time that sudden infant death syndrome has been under active investigation, numerous doctors have published the results of many series of cot deaths. From these, the constantly recurring features described in the first chapter of this book have emerged. Lists of things such as age, social class, season, twins, etc., have been collected assiduously and an almost constant pattern has emerged which has led to this form of death being recognised as a syndrome, rather than just a chance coming-together of similar features.

During the 1970s this process was taken much farther by several groups, especially those of Richard Naeye in the United States and John Emery and R. G. Carpenter in Great Britain. They analysed the epidemiological and sociological factors in many thousands of previous SIDS tragedies and picked out those which seemed to be associated with an increased risk of sudden, unexpected death. To say 'seemed to' is understating the case because they worked out probabilities and significance in a complex statistical way. Naeye's factors included eight features of pregnancy such as the presence of anaemia in the mother, how many cigarettes she smoked and whether there was protein in her urine – and 19 features in the new-born baby itself.

The other best-known survey was that carried out by Professor John Emery of Sheffield and Dr R. G. Carpenter of London, a medical statistician. They devised a scoring system to recognise the high-risk infant and applied it to a prospective survey – they looked at a group of babies and tried to identify what made particular infants die unexpectedly – rather than a retrospective series which can only use post-mortem data. (Interested readers can look up this survey in the relevant journals, i.e. those at positions 5 and 6 in the list of articles on page 159.)

Other screening measures have been, and are being employed, using not only the history from the medical records of the birth and the family but actual hard data from heart beat tracings at birth and even fetal tracings during pregnancy. These have not tallied with the risk of SIDS later on, neither has the PSA (prolonged sleep apnoea) index yet been proved to be related to the later risk of sudden infant death.

In conclusion, there is no reliable way at present either to predict SIDS or to prevent it. Though energetic research goes on continuously and with increasing fervour now that the attention of expert cardiorespiratory physiologists has been drawn into the problem, we have to accept the fact that the only sensible course of action at the moment is to adhere meticulously to the best standard of accepted medical care for the mother during pregnancy and for the infant in the first year of life. It is significant that the lowest SIDS rates seem to be in countries like Finland which has the best standard of ante- and post-natal care.

Leaflets and literature available on SIDS

A number of the organisations whose addresses are listed on pages 163–165 now provide a wide range of leaflets suitable not only for bereaved parents and families but also for all health care workers including doctors. Earlier in this book the texts of leaflets specifically written for the general practitioner and the casualty department of hospitals, have been reproduced in full. (These are leaflets issued by the Foundation for the Study of Infant Deaths and are reproduced with their permission.)

One leaflet issued by the Foundation for the Study of Infant Deaths concerns infant care guidance and is produced for mothers who are particularly worried after the loss of a previous baby. It is printed on stiff card with a hole enabling it to be hung up in a convenient place in the kitchen, nursery or near the telephone. It has a space for the telephone number of the GP. The text of the leaflet is as follows:

Infant Care Guidance

Feeding
Breast feeding is the natural and the best way to feed your baby. Coughs and colds and tummy upsets are less frequent in breast-fed babies because breast milk helps them to resist and recover from infection. The early months of breast feeding are the most valuable. You and your baby will succeed best if you are quiet and undisturbed when feeding.

If you cannot breast feed or if you decide at some time to change to bottle feeding, keep the bottle and teats sterilised.

Use a recommended baby milk up to the age of 6 months.

Follow the instructions for making up the feeds accurately and carefully. If your bottle fed baby appears hungry, the amount given at each feed and/or the number of feeds can be increased, but do not strengthen the mixture by adding extra milk powder. Never leave a baby sucking at his bottle on his own.

Very few babies need solid foods before the age of 3 months, but most want a mixed diet as well as milk feeds by the age of 6 months. Consult your health visitor or doctor about feeding and vitamin supplements.

Babies aged over 1 month are sometimes thirsty and want a drink of water (without sugar), which has been boiled once only and cooled. This is especially important if they are feverish or have a cold, a chest infection, diarrhoea or vomiting. Illness is hardly ever caused by teething.

Crying

All healthy babies cry from time to time; some babies cry much more than others and some babies cry regularly at a certain time of day. If crying continues and is not due to the usual causes— hunger, thirst, discomfort, wet or soiled nappies, tiredness, loneliness or being too hot or cold—and gentle rocking of the pram or cot, or cuddling does not settle the baby, then see your doctor or health visitor.

Sleeping position

Select a cot with a firm, well-fitting mattress; a baby does not need a pillow. Traditionally, new-born babies were put on their side to sleep with the lower elbow a little in front of the body and put down on the opposite side after the next feed; this is still good practice. A rolled nappy placed by the back will prevent the baby rolling onto his back. Some babies like to sleep on their tummy with the head turned on one side. As the baby grows, the position in which he or she settles happily is probably the best.

Temperature

Keep your young baby's room at an even temperature of about 65°F (19°C) both day and night. Newborn babies need to be well wrapped until about one month old after which they are better at keeping themselves warm. Protect your baby including his head from draughts and use the pram hood in chill winds. In cold weather a baby can lose heat quickly even in his cot or pram. To check whether your baby is warm enough put your hand beneath the covers to feel his body. If the room is too warm or the baby overclothed, a baby can get too hot; he will feel hot or sweaty to the touch and may be thirsty. Fresh air is good for healthy babies but not when he has a cold, or in foggy or cold weather. In hot weather keep the pram hood down and shade your sleeping baby from direct sunlight with a sun canopy.

Some Suggestions When to Consult a Doctor About Your Baby

If you think your baby is ill even without any obvious symptoms *contact* your doctor.

If your baby shows any of the following symptoms especially if he has more than one *your doctor* would expect you to ask for advice.

Always urgent
- a fit or convulsion, or turns blue or very pale
- quick, difficult or grunting breathing
- exceptionally hard to wake or unusually drowsy or does not seem to know you

Sometimes serious
- croup or a hoarse cough with noisy breathing
- cannot breathe freely through his nose
- cries in an unusual way or for an unusually long time or you think your baby is in severe pain
- refuses feeds repeatedly, especially if unusually quiet
- vomits repeatedly
- frequent loose motions especially if watery (diarrhoea) Vomiting and diarrhoea together can lead to excessive loss of fluid from the body and this may need urgent treatment
- unusually hot or cold or floppy

Even if you have consulted a doctor, health visitor or nurse, *if baby* is not improving or is getting worse, *tell your doctor again the same day.*

Emergency Action: Get Medical Help Immediately

- contact your doctor
- telephone for an ambulance (dial 999) or
- take the baby to a Hospital Accident or Casualty department

While waiting for a doctor or ambulance to arrive:

If baby is not breathing
- stimulate baby by flicking the soles of his feet or picking him up. If no response, begin *resuscitation* through his mouth and nose

- place baby on his back on a table or other firm surface
- suck his nose clear

If the baby does not gasp or breathe
- support the back of his neck, tilt his head backwards and hold his chin upwards
- open your mouth wide and breathe in
- seal your lips round his nose and mouth
- breathe *gently* into his lungs until his chest rises
- remove your mouth to allow the air to come out and let his chest fall
- repeat gentle inflations a little faster than your normal breathing rate, removing your mouth after each breath

Baby should begin to breathe within a minute or two

For a fit or convulsion
- lay your baby on his tummy with his head low and turned to one side
- clear his nose and mouth of any sick or froth
- if he is hot, cool by sponging his head with tepid water (just warm)

For a burn or scald
- put the burnt or scalded part immediately in clean cold water
- lightly cover the part with a very clean cloth or sterile dressing
- do not apply oil or ointments; do not prick blisters

For an accident
- give First Aid if you know how
- if your baby has swallowed pills, medicines or household liquids . . . *take the bottle to hospital as well*

Suggested further reading

United Kingdom

ARTICLES

Bonser, R., Knight, B. and West, R. (1978). Sudden infant death syndrome in Cardiff, association with epidemic influenza and temperature, 1955–1974. *International Journal of Epidemiology*, **7**, 335.

Battye, J. and Deakin, M. (1979). Surveillance reduces baby deaths. *Nursing Mirror*, 24 July.

Caddell, J. (1972). Magnesium deprivation in sudden unexpected infant death. *Lancet*, **2**, 258.

Carpenter, R. G. and Emery, J. (1974). Identification and follow-up of infants at risk of sudden death in infancy. *Nature*, **250**, 729.

Carpenter, R. G. and Emery, J. (1977). Final results of study of infants at risk of sudden death. *Nature*, **268**, 724.

Carpenter, R. G., Gardner, A., McWeeny, P. and Emery, J. (1977). Multi-stage scoring system for identifying infants at risk of unexpected death. *Archives of Disease in Childhood*, **52**, 606.

Carpenter, R. G. et al (1979). Identification of some infants at immediate risk of dying unexpectedly and justifying intensive study. *Lancet*, **2**, 343.

Chambers, D. R. (1973). Sudden and unexpected death in infancy. *Health Visitor*, **46**, 334.

Cooke, R. T. and Welch, R. G. (1964). A study in cot death. *British Medical Journal*, 1549.

Editorial (1978). Sleep apnoea in children. *British Medical Journal*, 1506. (10 June).

Emery, J. (1972). Welfare of families of children found unexpectedly dead. *British Medical Journal*, 612. (4 March)

Emery, J. (1973). Unexpected deaths in infancy. *Nursing Times*, 12 April.

Emery, J. (1973). The unexpected child death. *Midwives Chronicle and Nursing Notes*, May number.

Emery, J. (1976). Cot deaths and the health visitor. *Johnson's Baby Newsline*, Issue 4, Autumn.

Emery, J. (1976). Post-neonatal mortality in Sheffield. *Proceedings of the Royal Society of Medicine*, **69**, 338.

Emery, J. (1977). The pattern of child health today and its relation to the community. *Journal of the Institute of Health Education*, **15**, 2.

Emery, J. (1979). Cot death. *Journal of Maternal and Child Health*, **4**, 10. (October)

Froggatt, P., Lynes, M. A. and McKenzie, G. (1971). Epidemiology of sudden unexpected death in infancy in Northern Ireland. *British Journal of Preventive and Social Medicine*, **25**, 3.

Knight, B. (1971). Cot deaths. *Modern Mother*, May/June, 65.

Knight, B. (1972). Legal and administrative problems in the cot death syndrome. *Journal of the Forensic Science Society*, **12**, 581.

Leading article (1975). Cot death. *Lancet*, 1024.

Leading article (1979). Apnoea and unexpected child death. *Lancet*, 339. (18 August)

Leading article (1980). Sudden infant death syndrome and ventilatory control. *British Medical Journal*, **6236**, 337.

Limerick, Lady (1976). Support and counselling needs of families following a cot death bereavement. *Proceedings of the Royal Society of Medicine*, **69**, 839.

Limerick, Lady and Downham, M. A. P. S. (1978). Support for families bereaved by cot death: joint voluntary and professional view. *British Medical Journal*, 1527. (10 June)

Limerick, Lady (1979). Counselling parents who have lost an infant. *Journal of the Royal College of Physicians*, **13**, 4, 242.

Limerick, Lady (1979). Counselling parents who have experienced a cot death in their family. *Journal of Maternal and Child Health*, **4**, 11. (November)

McWeeny, P. (1977). The use of child care services related to sudden death in infancy. *Journal of the Institute of Health Education*, **15**, 2.

Mason, J. K., Harkness, R. A., Elton, R. A. and Bartholomew, S. (1980). Cot deaths in Edinburgh: Infant feeding and socio-economic factors. *Journal of Epidemiology and Community Health*, **34**, 35.

Moore, A. (1976). The cot death syndrome. *Midwife, Health Visitor and Community Nurse*, **12**, 5, 154.

Murphy, J. F., Newcombe, R. G. and Sibert, J. R. (1982). The epidemiology of sudden infant death syndrome. *Journal of Epidemiology and Community Health*, **36**, 17.

Office of Population Censuses and Surveys (1980). *Sudden infant death syndrome 1971–1978*; ref DH3 80/3, issued 2 December. HMSO, London.

Palmer, S. R., Wiggins, R. D. and Bewley, B. R. (1980). Infant deaths in inner London: A health care planning study. *Community Medicine*, **2**, 102.

Parish, W. E. et al (1960). Hypersensitivity to milk and sudden death in infancy. *Lancet*, 1106.

Report of a Working Party for Early Childhood Deaths in Newcastle (1977). Newcastle survey of deaths in early childhood 1974/76 with special reference to sudden unexpected deaths. *Archives of Disease in Childhood*, **52**, 828.

Sunderland, R., Worsman, S. and Variend, S. (1982). Management of sudden death in childhood. *Maternal and Child Health*, **5**, 166.

Teare, D. and Knight, B. (1971). Death in the cot. *Science Journal*, **7**, 71.

Valman, H. B. (1977). Cot death. *Update*, January.

Vesselinova-Jenkins, C. K. (1980). Model of persistent fetal circulation and sudden infant death syndrome (SIDS). *Lancet*, **2**, 8199, 831.

BOOKS

Camps, F. E. and Carpenter, R. G. (eds) (1972). *Sudden and Unexpected Deaths in Infancy (Cot Deaths)*. (Proceedings of the Cambridge Symposium.) John Wright and Sons Ltd, Bristol.

Emery, J. (1976). *Unexpected death in infancy. Early recognition of the at-risk situation*. In *Recent Advances in Paediatrics*, pp. 203–20 (ed Hull, D.). Churchill Livingstone, Edinburgh.

United States of America

ARTICLES

Bergman, A. B., Beckwith, J. B. and Ray, C. G. (1975). The apnea monitor business. *Pediatrics*, **56**, 1.

Steinschneider, A. (1976). A re-examination of the apnea monitor business. *Pediatrics*, **58**, 1.

Valdes-Dapena, M. et al (1968). Sudden unexpected death in infancy: A statistical analysis of certain socio-economic factors. *Journal of Pediatrics* (St Louis), **73**, 387.

Valdes-Dapena, M. (1977). Sudden unexplained infant deaths, 1970 through 1975: An evolution in understanding. *Pathology Annual*, **12**, 177.

Valdes-Dapena, M. (1981). Sudden infant death syndrome: a review of the medical literature 1974–1979. *Pediatrics*, **66**, 597.

BOOKS

Bergman, A. B., Beckwith, J. B. and Ray, C. G. (eds) (1970). *Sudden Infant Death Syndrome*. (Proceedings of the Second International Conference on SIDS, Seattle, 1979.) University of Washington Press.

Geertinger, P. (1966). *Sudden Death in Infancy*. Charles Thomas, Springfield, Ill.

Robinson, R. (ed) (1975). *'SIDS 1974'*. (Proceedings of the Toronto Symposium, 1974.) Canadian Foundation for the Study of Infant Deaths.

Wedgwood and Benditt (eds) (1964). *Sudden Death in Infancy*. (Proceedings of the Conference in Seattle, September 1963.) US Department of Health, Education and Welfare, NICHHD (NIH), Bethesada, Maryland.

Useful organisations

United Kingdom

The Foundation for the Study of Infant Deaths
5th Floor, 4 Grosvenor Place
London SW1X 7HD   01-235 1721 and 01-245 9421

The Compassionate Friends
5 Lower Clifton Hill
Bristol BS8   Bristol (0272) 292778

United States of America

SIDS Clearing House
1555 Wilson Boulevard, Suite 600
Rosslyn, VA 22209-2461   (703) 522-0870

National Sudden Infant Death Syndrome Foundation
(NSIDSF)
2 Metro Plaza, Suite 205
8240 Professional Place
Landover, Maryland 20785

International Council for Infant Survival (ICIS)
c/o Nina Copp, President
2956 Eric Lane
Dallas, Texas 75234

Australia

AUSTRALIA CAPITAL TERRITORIES
SID Association (ACT) Inc
PO Box 58, Jamison
ACT 2614   58 7509

NEW SOUTH WALES

SID Association of NSW
PO Box 172, St Ives
Sydney 2075   534 9045

QUEENSLAND

Queensland SID Research Foundation
The Secretary, PO Box 1987
Brisbane 4001   370 1311

SOUTH AUSTRALIA

SIDS Association of South Australia Inc
PO Box 114, Nodbury North
South Australia 5092   337 9688

TASMANIA

c/o Mrs M. Ballen
109 Howick Street
Launceston, Tasmania   31 3806 (W); 44 1905 (H)

c/o Dr Colin Hinrichsen
GPO Box 370
Hobart, Tasmania 7001   23 0561 (W)

VICTORIA

SID Research Foundation
283 Wattletree Road
East Malvern, Melbourne 3145   509 7722

WESTERN AUSTRALIA

SIDS Foundation
c/o Mr F. Watson (Vice-President)
219 Hamilton Street
Queens Park   451 4607

Canada

Canadian Foundation for the Study of Infant Death
181 Belsize Drive
Toronto, Ontario M4S 1L9

New Zealand

Cot Death Division,
National Children's Health Research Foundation
c/o Mrs A. McDonald
668 Remuera Road
Remuera, Auckland 5

South Africa

Cot Death Society
c/o Mrs J. Marais
PO Box 11306
Vlaeberg 8012

Index